Obstetric Decisions

This is a practical manual on troubleshooting options when there are obstetric complications, so medical staff can check quickly and easily on the essential points they need to know, do, and recommend.

Key Features:

- Offers a quick and easy-to-consult reference for essential points
- Presents an invaluable guide for those in training who need to make a decision in complicated circumstances
- Summarises its points in boxes, flow-charts, and tables

Obstetric Decisions
Quick Thinking for Safe Deliveries

Rhianna Davies, BSc (Hons), MBBS, PhD,
MRCOG, MIMP, DFMS, PGCE

Senior Registrar in Obstetrics and Gynaecology and Clinical
Research Fellow, Imperial College NHS Foundation Trust,
London, UK

Kelsie Sykes, BMBS, BMedSci,
MA(MedEd), MRCOG

Consultant Obstetrician, Mid and South Essex NHS Trust,
Basildon, UK

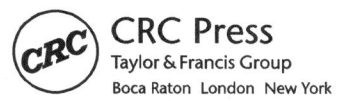

CRC Press
Taylor & Francis Group
Boca Raton London New York

CRC Press is an imprint of the
Taylor & Francis Group, an **informa** business

Designed cover image: Shutterstock

First edition published 2026
by CRC Press
2385 NW Executive Center Drive, Suite 320, Boca Raton FL 33431

and by CRC Press
4 Park Square, Milton Park, Abingdon, Oxon, OX14 4RN

CRC Press is an imprint of Taylor & Francis Group, LLC

ISBN: 9781032831718 (hbk)
ISBN: 9781032825229 (pbk)
ISBN: 9781003508151 (ebk)

DOI: 10.1201/9781003508151

Typeset in Times
by KnowledgeWorks Global Ltd.

Contents

Abbreviations

ABG	Arterial blood gas
AC	Abdominal circumference
ACIi	ACEi -Angiotensin-converting enzyme inhibitors
ACR	Albumin-creatinine ratio
AFE	Amniotic fluid embolism
AN	Antenatal
ANC	Antenatal clinic
APH	Antepartum haemorrhage
AP diameter	Anterior-posterior diameter
Apgar score	(score to evaluate health of all newborns at 1 and 5 minutes after birth and in response to resuscitation)
AREDV	Absent or reversed end-diastolic volume
ARDS	Acute respiratory distress syndrome
ARM	Artificial rupture of membranes
ART	Assisted reproductive techniques
BA	Bile acids
BG	Blood gas
BHIVA	British HIV Association
BM	Blood glucose level
BMI	Body mass index
cART	combined anti-retroviral therapy
Cat 1	Category 1
CCT	Controlled cord traction
cCTG	Continuous cardiotocography
cEFM	Continuous external fetal monitoring
CLC	Consultant led care
CLU	Consultant-led unit
CPD	Cephalo-pelvic disproportion
CPR	Cardiopulmonary resuscitation
C/S	Caesarean section
CSE	Combined spinal epidural
CSF	Cerebro-spinal fluid
CT	Computed tomography
CTG	Cardiotocography
D+V	Diarrhoea and vomitting
DIC	Disseminated intravascular coagulation
DCC	Delayed cord clamping
DDAVP	Desmopressin
DM	Diabetes mellitus

E+D	Eating and drinking
ECV	External cephalic version
EFM	External fetal monitoring
EFW	Estimated fetal weight
El C/S	Elective caesarean section
Em C/S	Emergency caesarean section
ERCS	Elective repeat caesarean section
ESBL	Extended spectrum beta-lactamase
FBC	Full blood count
FBS	Fetal blood sampling
FD	Fetal distress
FFN	Fetal fibronectin
FFP	Fresh frozen plasma
FHR	Fetal heart rate
FSE	Fetal scalp electrode
G+S	Group and save
GAS	Group A streptococcus
GBS	Group B streptococcus
GDM	Gestational diabetes mellitus
GI tract	Gastrointestinal tract
GT	Gestational thrombocytopenia
GTG	Green top guideline
GTT	Glucose tolerance test
GUM	Genito-urinary medicine
HAART	Highly active anti-retroviral therapy
HDU/ITU	High-dependency unit/intensive care unit
HTN	Hypertension
HSV	Herpes simplex virus
HVS	High vaginal swab
IA	Intermittent oscillation
ICP	Intrahepatic cholestasis of pregnancy
IM	Intramuscular
Index pregnancy	Current pregnancy
IOL	Induction of labour
IPV	Internal podalic version
IR	Interventional radiology
ITP	Idiopathic thrombocytopenic purpura
IUD	Intrauterine death
IUGR	Intrauterine growth restriction
IUT	In-utero transfer
IV	Intravenous
IVF	In vitro fertilisation
LA	Local anaesthetic
LFGA	Large for gestational age
LFT	Liver function tests

LGA	Large for gestational age
LLETZ	Large loop excision of transformation zone
LMWH	Low-molecular-weight heparin
LSCS	Lower section caesarean section
LUS	Lower uterine segment
LV	Liquor volume
LVS	Low vaginal swab
LW	Labour ward
MC + S	Microscopy, culture and sensitivity
MDT	Multi-disciplinary team
MEOWS	Modified Early Obstetric Warning Score
MgSO$_4$	Magnesium sulphate
MI	Myocardial infarction
MLC	Midwifery-led care
MLU	Midwife-led unit
MOH	Massive obstetric haemorrhage
MROP	Manual removal of placenta
MRSA	Methicillin-resistant Staphylococcus aureus
MSU	Mid-stream urine
MSV	Mauriceau Smellie-Veit
Multip	Multiparous woman
NEC	Necrotising enterocolitis
NICE	National Institute of Clinical Excellence
NICU	Neonatal intensive care unit
NIEL	Not in established labour
NIPT	Non-invasive prenatal testing
NVD	Normal vaginal delivery
NSAID	Non-steroidal anti-inflammatory drug
OA	Occipito-anterior
OASI	Obstetric anal sphincter injury
OP	Occipital-posterior
OT	Occipito-transverse
OVD	Operative vaginal delivery
PAS	placenta accreta spectrum
PDS	Polydioxanone suture
PE	Pulmonary embolism
PEA	Pulseless electrical activity
PET	Pre-eclamptic toxaemia
PEP	Post-exposure prophylaxis
PCI	Percutaneous intervention
PCR	Protein-creatinine ratio
PG	Prostaglandin
PIH	Pregnancy-induced hypertension
PN	Postnatal
PND	Postnatal depression

PP	Post-partum
PPE	Personal protective equipment
PPH	Post-partum haemorrhage
PPROM	Preterm prelabour rupture of membranes
Primip	Primiparous woman (first pregnancy)
PROM	Prelabour rupture of membranes
PT/APTT	Prothrombin time/activated partial thromboplastin time
PTB	Preterm birth
PTL	Preterm labour
PUR	Postnatal urinary retention
PV	Per vaginal
PVL	Panton-Valentine leukocidin
QDS	Four times per day
RA	Regional anaesthesia
RCOG	Royal College of Obstetricians and Gynaecologists
Reg	Registrar
RFM	Reduced fetal movements
ROM	Rupture of membranes
RPOC	Retained products of conception
SB	Still birth
SCBU	Special care baby unit
SD	Shoulder dystocia
SGA	Small for gestational age
SOB	Shortness of breath
SpR	Specialty registrar
SROM	Spontaneous rupture of membranes
Sx	Symptoms
Steroids	Corticosteroids, in this context
STI	sexually transmitted infection
Synto	Syntocinon (oxytocin augmentation)
TED	Thrombo-embolic disease
TENS	Transcutaneous electrical nerve stimulation
TORCH	Toxoplasmosis, Other infections, Rubella, Cytomegalovirus (CMV), and Herpes simplex virus (HSV).
TPTL	Threatened preterm labour
TV US	Transvaginal ultrasound scan
TXA	Tranexamic acid
U+Es	Urea and electrolytes
UAD	Umbilical artery doppler
US	Ultrasound
USS	Ultrasound scan
TWOC	Trial without catheter
VBAC	Vaginal birth after caesarean
VBG	Venous blood gas
VE	Vaginal examination
VF	Ventricular fibrillation

VT	Ventricular tachycardia
VTE	Venous thromboembolism
VWD	Von-Willebrands disease
VWF	Von-Willebrand factor
VZV	Varicella zoster virus
X-matched	Cross matched
Yo	Years old

1

The Management of the Latent Phase of Labour

Uncomplicated Latent Phase

From onset of contractions to 4 cm cervical dilatation.

Definition: A period of time, not necessarily continuous, when women experience painful contractions which may be associated with cervical changes, including effacement and dilation up to 4 cm.

The latent phase is a normal part of labour but of variable and unpredictable duration.

Assessment

- Professional discretion dictates whether or not a vaginal examination (VE) is indicated.
- Establish she has appropriate social support.
- If the woman is found to be in the latent phase and all clinical findings are within normal limits, advise her to return home.

Advice

- Adopt positions that promote fetal head rotation (e.g. standing, leaning forward, all fours).
- Strategies to manage pain include immersion in water, simple analgesia and TENS machine (RCOG).

If additional analgesia is required, opiate analgesia can be considered.

- Remain in hospital.
- Conduct hourly observations.
- If after 4–6 hours the woman remains in the latent phase of labour and is able to cope, she can return home if all clinical observations are normal.

DOI: 10.1201/9781003508151-1

Prolonged Latent Phase

- There is no standard definition for a prolonged latent phase of labour.
- The Royal College of Obstetricians and Gynaecologists (RCOG) says the latent phase can commonly last 18–24 hours.
- Malpositions may lead to prolonged latent phase.

Escalation for obstetric review if:

- A patient recurrently presents in latent phase, even in the presence of normal maternal and fetal wellbeing
- Fetal distress
- Maternal exhaustion
- Maternal pyrexia
- Maternal tachycardia
- Maternal dehydration
- Failure of descent of the presenting part or failure of cervical dilation despite, regular uterine contractions

Artificial rupture of membranes (ARM) +/− Syntocinon (oxytocin augmentation) (Synto) can be considered, if possible, with consultant review, but the patient must be aware of the implications on labour.

Induction of Labour

General principles are as follows (see **Figures 1.1** and **1.2**):

- *Prostaglandins* (*PGs*): Once labour is established, intermittent auscultation is recommended. Continuous fetal monitoring is not recommended in the absence of other risk factors.
- Since intermittent monitoring is acceptable after normal initial cardiotocography (CTG), labour in water is an option for induction of labour (IOL).
- Do not give Prostin until 24 hours post Propess.
- Do not start oxytocin until more than six hours has passed since PG administration due to combined uterotonic effect.
- Do not give oxytocin until 30 minutes have passed post-ARM and there is no evidence of cord prolapse or hyperstimulation.
- Offer an epidural to women in labour receiving oxytocin.
- Discuss analgesia prior to starting IV oxytocin as it will probably be more painful.
- Continuous CTG is recommended during oxytocin induction to observe for uterine hypercontractility (tachysystole or hyperstimulation) and fetal heart rate concerns.

- Oxytocin rate should be increased at 30-minute intervals, aiming to use the minimum dose possible to achieve four to five contractions in ten minutes.
- Generally, if not in established labour (NIEL) after 12 hours of oxytocin, then a full obstetric review should be conducted and a caesarean birth considered.

Following insertion of prostaglandin (Propess or Prostin)

- CTG 20 minutes pre insertion
- Continuous external fetal monitoring (cEFM) 1-hour post-insertion
- Eating and drinking (E+D) as normal
- Monitoring as per local guidelines based on risk
- If Propess falls out within 18 hours of insertion, it should be either reinserted or replaced with a new one; if Propess falls out over 18 hours post-insertion, then a vaginal examination should be performed to assess appropriateness of ARM

Following ARM

- *Primiparous woman* (*primip*): perform ARM followed by immediate instigation of oxytocin
- *Multiparous woman* (*multip*): perform ARM and allow two hours for spontaneous onset of contractions. If not contracting regularly at two hours, commence oxytocin.
- Re-examine four hours after the onset of regular contractions (for both primips and multips).

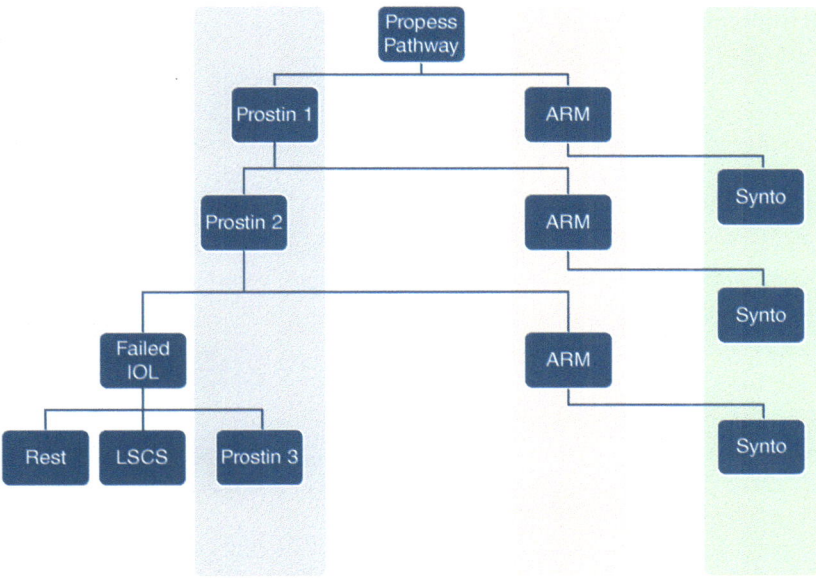

FIGURE 1.1 Management algorithm for insertion of prostaglandin.

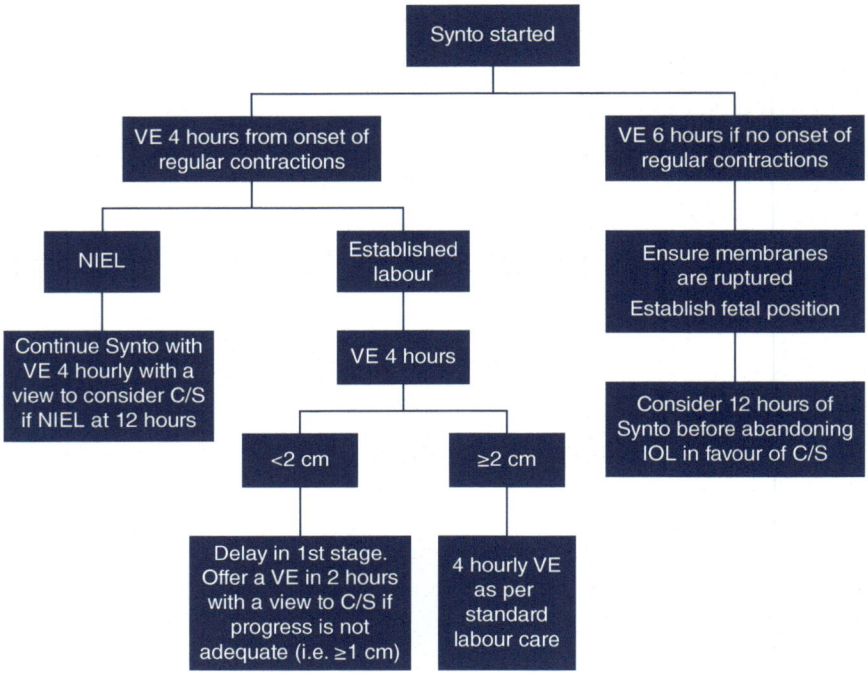

FIGURE 1.2   Management algorithm after starting oxytocin.

IOL in Special Circumstances

Induction of Labour Following PROM

Suggested regime: 1x Prostin → oxytocin (after six hours), or straight to oxytocin depending on Bishop's score on VE (immediate oxytocin if Bishop's Score >7)

There is evidence that further PG doesn't alter mode of delivery, but the additional time may increase the infection risk.

Handy tip: Have Prostin to hand when you perform the VE so that in the event the cervix is unfavourable and you elect to give it, you can administer immediately and avoid repeat examinations which will increase the risk of infection.

Induction of Labour for a Vaginal Birth after Caesarean

Discuss with consultant obstetrician.

PGs are contraindicated in the context of a vaginal birth after caesarean (VBAC). Mechanical induction methods with either Dilapan or a balloon catheter (depending on local protocols).

Suggested regime: Following ARM re-examine four hours after onset of regular contractions if using oxytocin, re-examine 2-hourly from then on.

LSCS indicated if:

1. NIEL after total twelve hours of oxytocin
2. Progress <2 cm at any one examination

Ineffective IOL

- If unable to ARM following full round of PG, offer the mother the following options:
  - Caesarean birth
  - Restarting IOL process after a 24-hour rest (if appropriate and maternal and fetal condition satisfactory on review)
- A difficult ARM in patient with an unfavourable cervix and no contractions, followed by oxytocin, is an option.
  - This is more likely to be successful in a multip.
  - Consider potential reasons for an unfavourable cervix in a multip, especially if there is fetal malposition, as there is an increased risk of uterine rupture if oxytocin is given with a malpositioned head.

CTG concerns during IOL

If you are called to review a patient with CTG concerns during IOL consider the following:

- Is this a prolonged bradycardia?

  *If so the usual 3-6-9-12 rule (see **Figure 1.3**) applies. Consider starting transfer to theatre early for caesarean section (C/S) as the patient is likely to be on the antenatal ward and unprepped for theatre. The C/S decision can always be stepped down if fetal bradycardia is resolved.*

- What has the CTG prior to this event been like?

  A normal CTG followed by a period of abnormality suggests the baby will have more reserves than a baby with a gradually declining CTG.

  Carefully assess the baseline fetal heart rate (FHR); a rising baseline is a suggestion of distress.

- Could this be part of a sleep cycle?

  Follow local CTG interpretation guidelines.

- What are maternal contractions like?

  Contracting > 4/10 + Abnormal CTG = Hyperstimulation; this requires intervention to reduce the frequency of contractions.

  Contracting > 4/10 + Normal CTG = Tachysystole; in the absence of CTG concerns the contractions do not need to be reduced urgently (but remain aware that if tachysystole persists, fetal distress may develop).

In the event of a CTG that you are concerned about, the following is advised:

- Take conservative measures of left lateral position and consider fluid replacement if hypovolaemia is suspected.
- Ensure at least one large-bore cannula, and consider FBC and group and save (G+S) in anticipation of an emergency C/S
- Examine the patient with a view to remove the prostaglandin if possible (Propess can be removed).
- If possible, perform an ARM – assess for the presence of meconium.

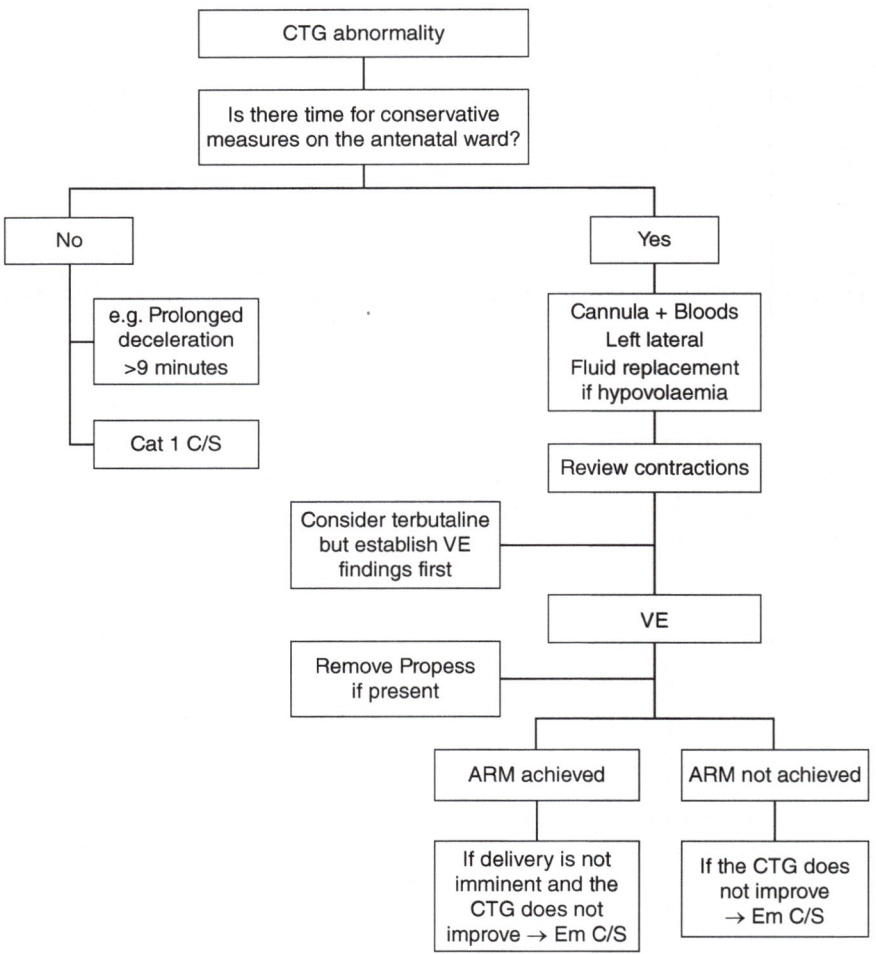

FIGURE 1.3   Management algorithm for CTG abnormality.

Terbutaline

- Consider terbutaline if hyperstimulating
- Terbutaline can be given to a patient with an abnormal CTG and contractions that don't exceed 4:10.
- Be aware terbutaline may give the baby a rest from contractions, but the contractions will return within 20–30 minutes and terbutaline increase the risk of bleeding.
- Do not give terbutaline prior to establishing VE findings. If she is fully dilated and delivery is imminent, advise pushing.

Troubleshooting: IOL Complications

If you are unable to ARM and the CTG subsequently normalises, allow 30 minutes of normal trace before restarting IOL. If you removed a Propess, insert the next only for a cumulative 24 hours.

It is preferable to have a patient who has had an abnormal CTG, even though it has normalised, on the labour ward in anticipation of it happening again. Therefore, transfer to the LW early, as either they will need expedited delivery, or they will be going there anyway once the CTG has resolved.

An emergency C/S can be stood down if the CTG normalises upon arrival. It is better to go to theatre early and for it to normalise than to go too late.

If the CTG normalises but meconium was found during ARM, manage as per all meconium in labour – offer expedition of labour with oxytocin. Allow at least 30 minutes of normal trace before starting it, and do not start if already hyperstimulating. If contracting, the mother can be given the option to await events; however, counsel that meconium can be a sign of distress and unnecessary delays in labour should be avoided.

2

The Management of the First Stage of Labour

Uncomplicated First Stage of Labour

From 4 cm to 10 cm

NICE (2014) recognises that the duration of active labour varies between women but suggests that

- First labours average 8 hours and are unlikely to last over 18 hours
- Second or subsequent labours average 5 hours and are unlikely to last over 12 hours

NICE (2014) recommendation for VEs:

- 4 hourly VEs in the first stage of labour
- VE in between these times only if there is concern about progress or at the woman's request
- Cervical dilatation 2 cm in 4 hours is considered reasonable normal progress (**Figure 2.1**)

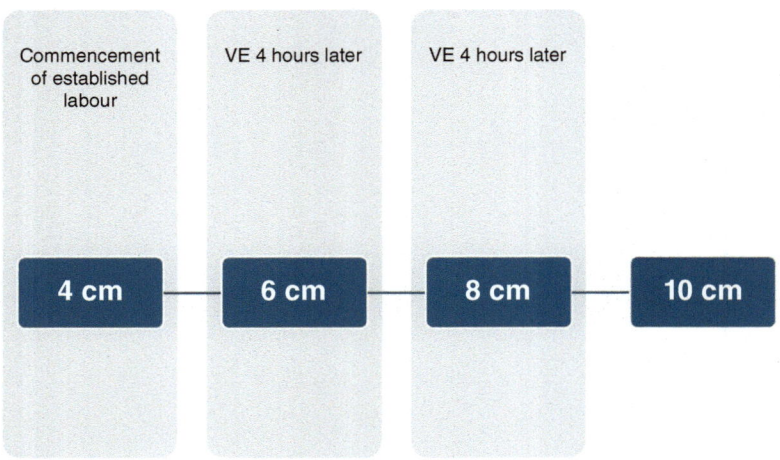

FIGURE 2.1   Reasonable progress of dilation in labour.

DOI: 10.1201/9781003508151-2

Delay in the First Stage (Table 2.1)

- **Suspect** delay if there is less than 2 cm progress in cervical dilation in 4 hours for primip and/or slowing in progress for a multip.
- Whether or not the woman accepts ARM at this point, NICE advise a follow-up VE after 2 hours.
- **Diagnose** delay if on 2-hour repeat, VE <1 cm progress in dilatation
- Start oxytocin
- Repeat VE after 4 hours
- C/S should be advised if one of the following three criteria is fulfilled:
  1. Oxytocin is contraindicated
  2. There is no further labour progress
  3. There are fetal heart rate concerns

See **Figure 2.2** for how to manage a delay in the first stage of labour.

TABLE 2.1

Causes of a Prolonged Labour

Fetal	Malposition or Malpresentation
Cephalo-pelvic disproportion (CPD)	Previous uncomplicated delivery of a baby of similar weight is the most reliable predictor of pelvic adequacy. CPD is suspected during labour if there is a lack of descent of the presenting part, often caput and moulding, slow progress from 7 cm onwards and slow second stage. Predisposing factors include maternal diabetes, a macrosomic baby or malposition. True CPD is not common.
Epidural	Epidural is associated with slow labour progress, increased malrotation and instrumental delivery secondary to labour dystocia from malposition.
Full bladder	Intermittent catheterisation is advised. Several randomised control trials have found indwelling catheter during the second stage is linked to delay; however, this is used if an epidural is in situ.
Denying or restricting food and fluids	Women who eat, drink and sleep well in the latent phase and preceding 24 hours tend to have shorter labours independent of other risk factors.
Emotional stresses	Increase catecholamine production (adrenaline) which may compete with oxytocin and inhibit contractions.

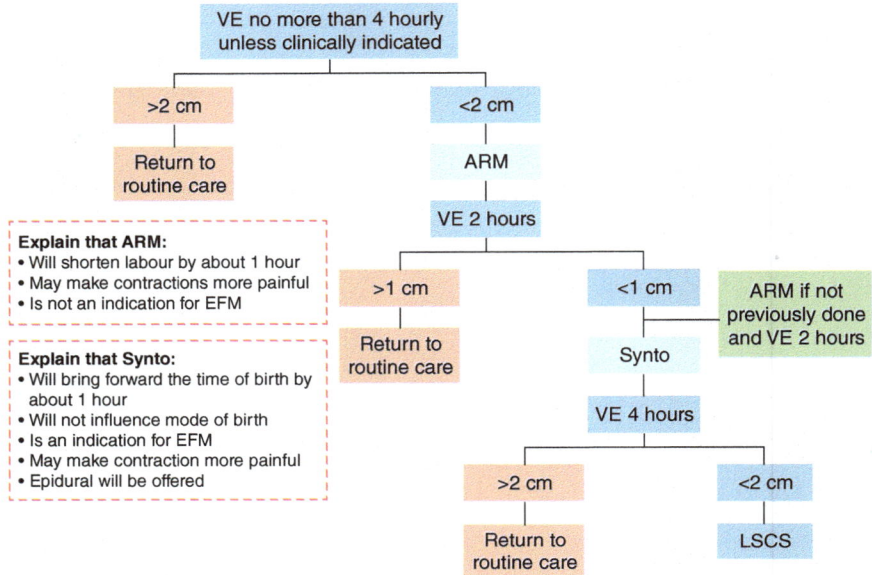

FIGURE 2.2   Management algorithm for delay in the first stage.

ARM

- NICE does not recommend the use of routine ARM
- NICE advises ARM for slow progress
- Repeat VE 2 hours post ARM

By far the most serious risk of ARM is cord prolapse leading to fetal hypoxia. More than 50% of cord prolapse occur following ARM, with a perinatal death rate of 91/1000. See **Boxes 2.1** and **2.2**.

BOX 2.1   RISKS OF ARM

Risk factors for cord prolapse include anything that results in a poorly fitting presenting part

1. Preterm labour
2. Grand multiparity
3. Malpresentation

BOX 2.2   CONTRAINDICATIONS TO ARM

1. Placenta praevia or low-lying placenta
2. High or mobile presenting part
3. Women with a STI/genital tract infection (ARM should be performed at least 4 hours after antibiotics in women who are GBS+ve)
4. Undiagnosed or untreated HIV positive women

Oxytocin

- Oxytocin shortens labour by approximately 1 hour but does not affect C/S or instrumental rate.
- While C/S rates may remain unchanged, the indications are different - oxytocin reduces C/S of slow progress but increases C/S for fetal distress.
- Oxytocin augmentation is an independent risk factor for obstetric anal sphincter injuries (OASI) even in spontaneous deliveries of normal sized infants.
- Women should be carefully observed for hyperstimulation and fetal heart rate concerns - NICE recommends continuous CTG.
- Oxytocin can be used in women having a vaginal birth after C/S, but the uterine rupture risk is increased, and so continuous monitoring is indicated, with a low threshold for C/S if concerns.

NB: Slow progress from 7 cm should be observed carefully.

Fetal Malposition and Malpresentation (Table 2.2)

TABLE 2.2

Fetal Presentations: First Stage of Labour

Lie	Presentation	Position	Management
Longitudinal	**VERTEX**	OA	Expectant
		OP	Expectant
		OT	• Expectant • Failure of the head to rotate during first stage leads to transverse arrest (requires rotation for vaginal delivery, or C/S if rotation unsuccessful).

(Continued)

TABLE 2.2 *(Continued)*

Fetal Presentations: First Stage of Labour

Lie	Presentation	Position	Management
Longitudinal	**BROW**		• Expectant – unstable position and tends to convert to vertex or face. Can't be delivered vaginally if persists. • There is increased adverse morbidity associated with a persistent brow presentation, e.g. fetal heart rate abnormalities, meconium-stained liquor and lower Apgar scores.
	FACE	Mento-anterior	• Expectant • There is increased adverse morbidity associated with a persistent face presentation, e.g. fetal heart rate abnormalities, meconium-stained liquor and lower Apgar scores.
		Mento-posterior	• Expectant • 30% will rotate to mento-anterior • Can't be delivered vaginally if persists
	BREECH	Complete Extended Footling Kneeling	• Planned breech delivery is covered in Chapter 6. • Unexpected breech presentation in labour can be managed either expectantly or by C/S in the event it is not advanced. • Planned C/S leads to small reducton in perinatal mortality compared with planned vaginal breech delivery: the risk of perinatal mortality is 0.5/1000 with C/S after 39+0 weeks of gestation; and approximately 2.0/1000 with planned vaginal breech birth. This compares to approximately 1.0/1000 with planned cephalic birth. Data for unplanned breech deliveries and intrapartum C/S for breech are lacking. • Routine C/S is not recommended in spontaneous preterm breech presentation. • Routine C/S is not recommended in spontaneous preterm breech presentation at the threshold of viability (22–25+6).

(Continued)

TABLE 2.2 *(Continued)*

Fetal Presentations: First Stage of Labour

Lie	Presentation	Position	Management
Transverse	**SHOULDER**		• Undeliverable vaginally • Em C/S • Risk of cord prolapse

Meconium

Significant meconium is defined by NICE as: 'dark green or black amniotic fluid that is thick or tenacious, or any meconium-stained amniotic fluid containing lumps of meconium'.

- Meconium-stained liquor may just represent a mature fetal GI tract (see **Box 2.3**)
- Meconium is rare <34/40
- In some cases, it can be associated with increased morbidity and mortality
- Aspiration into the baby's lungs during intrauterine gasping or once ex-utero can result in meconium aspiration syndrome which can be life threatening

BOX 2.3   RISK FACTORS FOR MECONIUM-STAINED LIQUOR

- Placental insufficiency
- Maternal hypertension and pre-eclampsia
- Oligohydramnios
- Smoking
- Substance misuse (particularly cocaine abuse)
- Increased maternal age
- Post 41 weeks gestation

Pre-Labour Meconium

Any woman who contacts maternity services reporting term pre-labour rupture of membranes with evidence of meconium must be invited in for review.

If meconium is confirmed:

- Senior review
- cEFM
- IOL advised - if meconium is present by definition ROM has occurred - IOL is achieved as described in chapter 1 for SROM

Meconium in Labour in the Community

- If significant meconium - ideally transfer to an obstetric unit (if safe to), as neonatal support may be needed

Intrapartum Care in the Presence of Meconium

- If meconium is identified in the MLU, transfer to CLU
- Alert senior midwife and on call obstetrician
- Confirm fetal presentation. THINK breech
- Advise cEFM due to association with meconium and fetal hypoxia
- Advise oxytocin augmentation to avoid delay in labour progress
- Paediatrician present at delivery
- If the baby is in good condition at birth delayed cord clamping can be performed as normal

Bladder Care

Intrapartum Care

- Women must be encouraged to pass urine at least every 4 hours during labour.
- A fluid balance chart must be kept where epidurals or IV fluid are in progress.
- **If ≥500 mLs is drained with an in/out catheter, an indwelling catheter should be inserted, and a fluid balance chart commenced.**

2nd Stage Bladder Care

- For delivery, catheter balloon must be deflated.
- If performing an instrumental delivery, the bladder must be emptied prior to placing of the instrument on the fetal head.
- If there has been urinary retention ≥700 mlLs in labour, catheterisation is advised for at least 24 hours postnatally.

Postnatal Care

- Once indwelling catheter is removed, voided volume should be assessed for a few hours.
- A fluid balance chart should be kept. This is reviewed for volume and timing of voids. Women must be asked if the void was normal for them, with normal sensation and perceived complete emptying.
- The woman must not be encouraged to drink large volumes of fluids too quickly following TWOC.

A void of ≥200 mLs with normal sensation suggests normal voiding.

Troubleshooting: Reduced Urine Output in Labour (Figure 2.3)

Fluid balance
- Review the fluid balance chart first. Recalculate the amount of fluid that has gone in and come out accurately.

Examination
- Examine the patient to make sure that the catheter is correctly placed.
- A low fetal head can be a cause of reduced urine output in the active phase of labour.

Investigation
- Remember that reduced urine output can be a manifestation of renal involvement in pre-eclampsia. Check renal function.

Management
- Consider giving a small fluid challenge (e.g. 250 ml) to help identify and treat volume depletion as a cause of the reduced urine output.

Reassess
- It is paramount that an assessment of response to the fluid challenge follows the administration.

FIGURE 2.3 Troubleshooting schedule for reduced urine output.

3

The Management of the Second Stage of Labour

Uncomplicated Second Stage

From full dilatation (10 cm) until the baby has been born:

- For a patient without an epidural: If she has no urge to push, she should wait 1 hour after confirmation that she is fully dilated.
- For a patient with an epidural: Delay pushing 1 hour after confirmation of full dilation unless the head is visible, or the woman has the urge to push.
- For a primip with inadequate contractions at the onset of the second stage consider oxytocin. Offer epidural anaesthesia if starting oxytocin.
- Perform vaginal examination (VE) after 1 hour of active second stage for a primip or after 30 minutes for a multip.
- Offer artificial rupture of membranes (ARM) if membranes are still intact.
- If birth is not imminent after 2 hours of active pushing in a primip or 1 hour in a multip, then obstetric review should be carried out every 15–30 minutes if there are no fetal well-being concerns (**Figures 3.1** and **3.2**).
- Birth should take place after 4 hours from fully dilated regardless of parity, inclusive of the 1 passive hour.

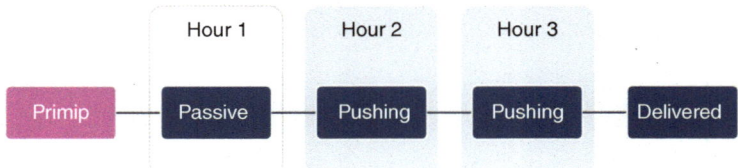

FIGURE 3.1   Reasonable schedule for primip.

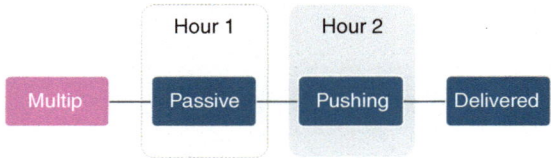

FIGURE 3.2   Reasonable schedule for multip.

                                         DOI: 10.1201/9781003508151-3

Slow Progress in the Second Stage (Table 3.1)

TABLE 3.1

Checklist for Slow Progress in the Second Stage

☐ Is the cervix fully dilated?
☐ Is the bladder full?
☐ Does she have a genuine urge to push if not, she could be experiencing a latent second phase of labour?
☐ Could the women change position or be more upright?
☐ Are the contractions adequate?

NICE define second stage delay as:

- *Primip*: 2 hours of active second stage. Instrumental delivery is advised after 3 hours (**Figure 3.3**).

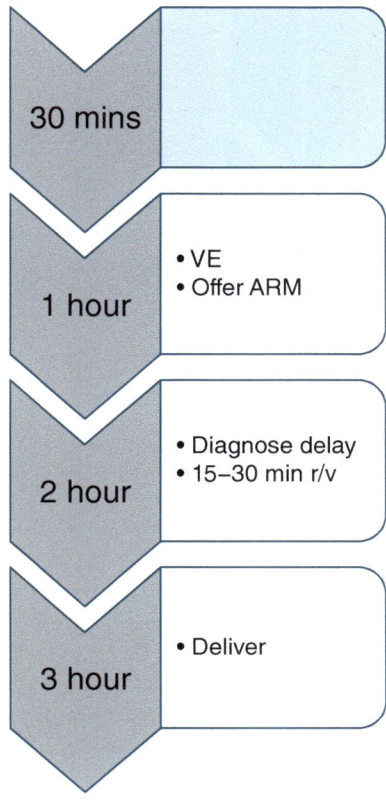

30 mins

1 hour
- VE
- Offer ARM

2 hour
- Diagnose delay
- 15–30 min r/v

3 hour
- Deliver

FIGURE 3.3 Reasonable schedule for primip.

- *Multip*: 1 hour active second stage. Instrumental delivery is advised after 2 hours (**Figure 3.4**).

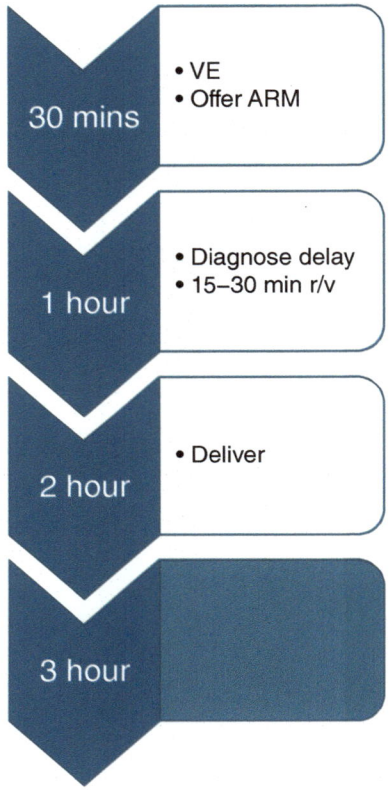

FIGURE 3.4   Reasonable schedule for multip.

- Birth within 4 hours whatever the parity.

NICE recommends

- Offering VE after an hour of active second stage for a primip or 30 minutes for a multip to assess rotation and descent.
- ARM if membranes are intact.
- If birth isn't imminent after 2 active hours for primip or 1 active hour for a multip, then an obstetric review should take place every 15–30 minutes if there are no fetal well-being concerns.
- Expedited delivery after 3 hours of active second stage for a primip, 2 hours of active second stage for a multip.

Troubleshooting: Expediting Delivery

☐ **Decide where and how to deliver**

- *Delivery method and location depend on the presence or absence of maternal or fetal compromise. In an otherwise uncomplicated delay in the 2nd stage there is time to transfer to theatre for a trial of instrumental delivery. Perform an instrumental delivery in the room only if you are absolutely sure it can be achieved; if in doubt, do it in theatre with the ability to convert to caesarean section (C/S). Fetal malposition or malpresentation may make attempts at vaginal delivery less successful (see **Table 3.1**).*

- *In the presence of fetal compromise, deliver via the quickest route. If delivery in the room is achievable, this is the fastest; however, be mindful that a failed delivery in the room and then conversion to a Cat 1 C/S takes longer than moving to theatre in the first instance.*

☐ **Anticipate complications**

- *Consider the possibility of delay in the 2nd stage being due to a larger baby and prepare for a possible shoulder dystocia.*

- *Anticipate a post-partum haemorrhage (PPH) following delivery associated with a delay in the 2nd stage of labour. Ask for prophylactic oxytocic at delivery (if no contraindications) +/− Syntocinon infusion.*

Table 3.2 shows fetal presentations in second stage of labour.

TABLE 3.2

Management of Fetal Malposition or Malpresentation in the Second Stage of Labour

Lie	Presentation	Position	Management
Longitudinal	**VERTEX**	Occipito-anterior (OA)	• Expectant
		Occipital-posterior (OP)	• Expectant • It is possible to spontaneously delivery an OP baby vaginally, especially in a multip • Attempt to rotate to OA and deliver with forceps • If unable to rotate, C/S
		Occipito-transverse (OT)	• Undeliverable vaginally • Attempt to rotate or C/S

(Continued)

TABLE 3.2 *(Continued)*

Management of Fetal Malposition or Malpresentation in the Second Stage of Labour

Lie	Presentation	Position	Management
Longitudinal	BROW		• Expectant – unstable position and tends to convert to vertex or face • Difficult to deliver vaginally • If persists, C/S
	FACE	Mento-anterior	• Expectant • Can be delivered vaginally • Do not apply FSE or ventouse
		Mento-posterior	• Expectant • 30% will rotate to mento-anterior • Can't be delivered vaginally • If persists, C/S
	BREECH	Complete Extended Footling Kneeling	• Planned breach delivery is covered in Chapter 6 • Routine C/S is not recommended in or near the 2nd stage of labour • If time permits, perform a US to establish the EFW, and position of the neck and legs to tailor counselling
Transverse	SHOULDER	Undeliverable vaginally	• Unlikely to reach fully dilated as no pressure on cervix from presenting part • More likely at FD if it is a 2nd twin – ECV or IPV + Breech extraction • Risk of cord prolapse

Abbreviations: ECV, external cephalic version; EFW, estimated fetal weight; FSE, fetal scalp electrode; IPV, internal podalic version; US, ultrasound.

4

The Management of the Third Stage of Labour

Uncomplicated Third Stage

The National Institute of Clinical Excellence (NICE) advises active management.

A woman with low post-partum haemorrhage (PPH) risk requesting physiological management can be supported.

Physiological vs Active Management

- Active management appears to reduce blood loss immediately following birth.
- Overall blood loss by hour 36 is similar with active or physiological management.
- Active management is quicker (5–10 minutes vs 20–60 minutes)
- A Cochrane review found active management increases the risk of readmission later with bleeding, and increases oxytocin side effects such as headache, nausea, vomiting, severe after pains.
- Neither method appears to have any significant adverse effects for the baby.

Active Management of Third Stage

- Give a prophylactic oxytocic after delivery of the anterior shoulder or following birth.
- Cochrane review suggested Syntometrine (ergometrine + oxytocin) reduces blood loss of 500–1000 mL more effectively than oxytocin alone but does not do so for blood losses of greater >1000 mL
- Syntometrine carries the side effects of hypertension, nausea and vomiting, and retained placenta due to cervical closing.
- NICE (2014) recommends IV Syntocinon 10 IU IM, stating fewer side effects compared with Syntometrine.

DOI: 10.1201/9781003508151-4

Prolonged Third Stage

- NICE (2014) defines prolonged third stage as an undelivered placenta after 30 minutes of active management.
- PPH risk increases after this time.
- It may be necessary to proceed to manual removal of the placenta (**Tables 4.1** and **4.2**).

TABLE 4.1

Risk Factors for a Retained Placenta

- Previous retained placenta
- Multiparity
- Maternal age > 35 years
- Induction of labour (IOL)
- Preterm labour (PTL)
- Placenta praevia+/−abnormally invasive placenta
- Uterine anomalies, e.g. bicornuate uterus, fibroids
- Previous uterine surgery or instrumentation

TABLE 4.2

Complications of a Retained Placenta

- PPH
- Shock
- Sepsis
- Perforation
- Retained products
- Uterine inversion
- Uterine, cervical, vaginal trauma
- Rhesus–isoimmunisation
- Anaesthetic complications
- Severe maternal morbidity and death

Management of Retained Placenta

- Alert the obstetric registrar if the placenta is not delivered within 30 minutes of active management or 60 minutes of physiological management + stable patient + no significant bleeding.
- Do not leave patient unattended.
- If unable to gently remove in the room, transfer to theatre for manual removal of placenta (MROP; **Table 4.3**, see further text in **Figure 4.1**).

TABLE 4.3

Potential complications of manual removal of placenta (MROP)

- Bleeding
- Infection
- Trauma to uterus, cervix, vagina
- Failure to remove all tissue
- Repeat procedure, return to theatre
- Balloon tamponade
- Blood transfusion
- Laparotomy
- Hysterectomy

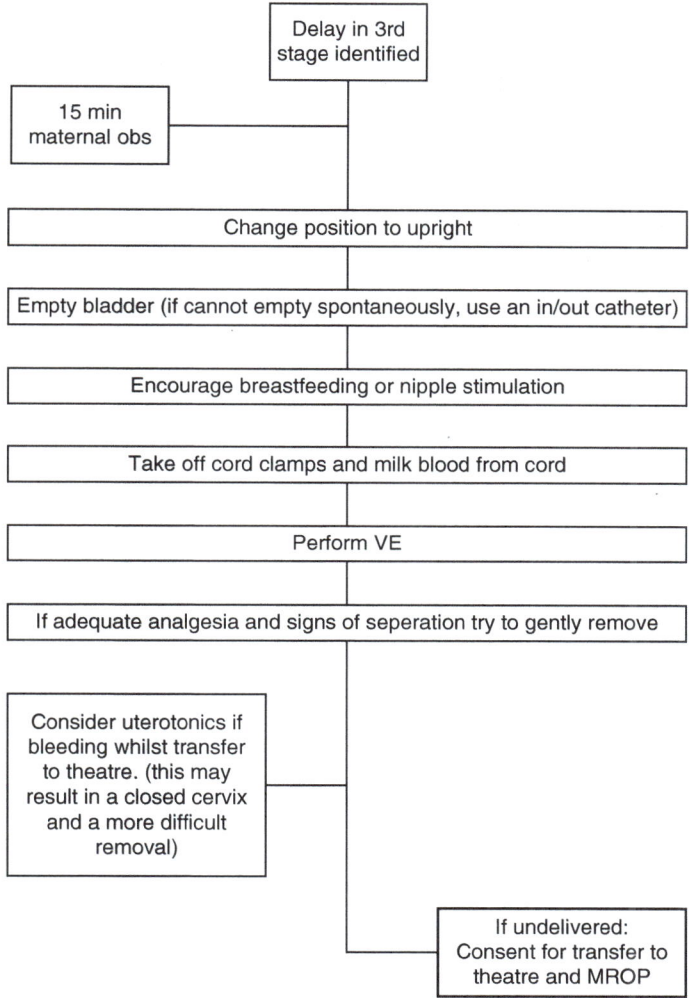

FIGURE 4.1 Management algorithm for delay in third stage.

Procedure of MROP

- Position patient appropriately with legs in lithotomy.
- Clean and drape.
- Ensure tested and adequate regional anaesthesia.
- Administer STAT IV antibiotic as per local guidelines (e.g. co-amoxiclav or clindamycin + gentamicin)

- Empty the bladder – insert indwelling catheter in light of regional anaesthesia.
- Stabilise fundus with non-dominant hand.
- Gently insert hand through cervix and identify the placental plane.
- If plane between placenta and uterus is not easily defined, consider placenta accreta and inform the on-call consultant. Do not pull on the cord or placenta.
- Using the side of your hand and a sweeping motion, sweep the placenta from the uterine wall.
- Guard the fundus to avoid uterine inversion.
- Grasp the uppermost portion of the placenta and aim to remove the whole placenta in one piece.
- Confirm the cavity is empty.
- Assess the placenta to ensure it is complete.
- Massage the uterus to induce contractions.
- Inspect for tears and repair as required.
- IV oxytocin infusion should commence (40 iu of oxytocin in 500 mL of sodium chloride over 4 hours) if active bleeding.

5

The General Principles of Intrapartum Care

Analgesia

Non-Pharmacological Analgesia

- *Aromatherapy*
- *Hypnosis and hypnotherapy*: Current available evidence shows that hypnosis reduces the need for pharmacological pain relief including regional analgesia.
- *TENS machines*: These are not recommended by the National Institute of Clinical Excellence (NICE) but anecdotally many women find them helpful
- *Deep water immersion* (i.e. water birth)
    - The Royal College of Obstetricians and Gynaecologists (RCOG; 2006) recommends that the opportunity to deliver in water should be available to all healthy women with uncomplicated pregnancies (**Tables 5.1** and **5.2**).
    - NICE (2014) states that the evidence supports water immersion in labour but does not prove or disprove the benefits of actual birth in water.
    - A Cochrane review (2018) reported overall low-quality evidence from which to draw conclusions but that water-immersion in labour probably results in fewer women having an epidural but probably makes little or no difference to the number of women who have a normal vaginal delivery (NVD), instrumental birth, caesarean section (C/S) or a serious perineal injury, or the number of babies admitted to neonatal intensive care unit (NICU) or developing infections.

TABLE 5.1

Criteria for Labouring in Water

1. Term pregnancy, i.e. ≥37 weeks
2. Singleton cephalic presentation
3. Labour appears uncomplicated and is progressing well
4. Reassuring maternal and fetal labour observations
5. Any opioid given more than 2 hours previously and woman is not drowsy
6. You can get waterproof cardiotocography (CTG) machines but someone requiring continuous monitoring might be better placed out of the pool for observation purposes, e.g. antepartum haemorrhage (APH)

DOI: 10.1201/9781003508151-5

TABLE 5.2

Contraindications to Water Birth

---

1. Pre-existing infection
2. Pyrexia
3. Prelabour rupture of membranes (PPROM)
4. Raised body mass index (BMI) (a relative contraindication)
5. A need for continuous monitoring in the absence of a waterproof monitor
6. Heavy bleeding or significant meconium liquor
7. Oxytocin augmentation
8. Previous C/S, i.e. vaginal birth after caesarean (VBAC)
9. Breech presentation

Pharmacological Analgesia

- *Entonox* (nitrous oxide)
  - It is short-acting.
  - There is no evidence of harm to the baby.
  - Maternal side effects are minor including dry mouth and nausea.
- *Opioids* (e.g. pethidine, diamorphine, meptazinol)
  - Maternal side effects include nausea and vomiting.
  - NICE recommends they be given with an anti-emetic.
  - Neonatal side effects include respiratory depression, subdued behaviour patterns, lack of responsiveness, drowsiness and reduced early breastfeeding.
  - Maternal side effects include nausea and vomiting.

Regional Analgesia/Anaesthesia

There are three options for regional analgesia/anaesthesia (RA):

1. *Epidural*: A catheter is inserted into the epidural space.
2. *Spinal*: Local anaesthetic is injected through the subarachnoid space into the cerebrospinal fluid. It is faster and shorter-acting than an epidural.
3. *Combined spinal epidural (CSE)*: A single spinal injection is given, plus an epidural catheter which remains in their back. It is faster acting than epidural but gives no better pain relief compared with an epidural alone.

NICE recommends low-dose bupivacaine (local anaesthetic) and fentanyl (opiate) for optimal labour outcomes and shows no preference for epidural vs CSE unless rapid regional anaesthesia is required (**Table 5.3**).

TABLE 5.3

Regional Anaesthesia in Women Taking Low-Molecular-Weight Heparin

Clinical Situation	Recommendation
Patient taking prophylactic dose LMWH	Last dose needs to be at least 12 hours prior to RA
Patient taking therapeutic dose LMWH	Last dose needs to be at least 24 hours prior to RA
Following regional anaesthesia	Wait at least 4 hours before administering LMWH
Epidural catheter removal	12 hours since last dose of LMWH 4 hours before next dose of LMWH

Requirements for RA

- IV access
- Blood pressure monitoring at 5-minute intervals for 15 minutes following establishment of the block or following a top up.
- CTG for at least 30 minutes at the establishment of the block or following top up.
- Regular rolling or movement of the women especially if raised BMI.
- Either an intermittent or indwelling urinary catheter.

Complications of RA

- Maternal hypotension
- Increased intervention – IV access, catheter, CTG
- Increased fetal malposition
- Increased need for oxytocin augmentation
- Urinary retention (reduced by low dose epidural)
- Prolonged second stage of labour
- Increased instrumental delivery rate
- Increased severe perineal trauma
- Increase fetal heart irregularities
- Increased C/S for fetal heart rate (FHR) concerns

Bladder Care

Intrapartum care

- Women must be encouraged to pass urine at least every 4 hours during labour.
- A fluid balance chart must be kept where epidurals or IV fluid are in progress.
- If ≥500 mL is drained with an in/out catheter, an indwelling catheter should be inserted, and a fluid balance chart commenced.

2nd stage bladder care

- For delivery, catheter balloon must be deflated.
- If performing an instrumental delivery, the bladder must be emptied prior to placing of the instrument on the fetal head.
- If there has been urinary retention ≥700 mL in labour, catheterisation is advised for at least 24 hours postnatally.

Postnatal care

- Once indwelling catheter is removed, voided volume should be assessed for the first two times that the woman passes urine.
- A fluid balance chart should be kept. This is reviewed for volume and timing of voids. Women must be asked if the void was normal for them, with normal sensation and perceived complete emptying.
- The woman must not be encouraged to drink large volumes of fluids too quickly following trial without catheter (TWOC).
- A void of ≥200 mL with normal sensation suggests normal voiding.

Eating and Drinking

- Pregnant women are at increased risk of inhalation of acidic gastric acid contents and associated complications (Mendelson's Syndrome).
- Therefore, patients at high risk (**Table 5.4**) of requiring a general anaesthetic require prophylaxis: clear fluids only + consider proton pump inhibitor once in active labour.
- The risk must be balanced against the risk of dehydration and ketosis in labour.

TABLE 5.4

Patients at High Risk of Requiring a General Anaesthetic in Labour

- Multiple pregnancy
- Abnormal presentation
- Placental abruption
- Previous lower section caesarean section (LSCS)
- Prolonged/slow progress in labour
- Epidural anaesthesia
- Induction of labour (IOL)/oxytocin augmentation
- Booking BMI >35

Fetal Heart Rate Monitoring in Labour

Intermittent Auscultation

Intermittent oscillation (IA) is recommended for low-risk pregnancies.

- IA should be done for 1 minute after a contraction every 15 minutes in the first stage of labour and every 5 minutes in the second stage of labour.
- If abnormalities in FHR are detected on IA (e.g. decelerations, bradycardia or tachycardia), NICE (2017) recommends carrying out more frequent auscultation (i.e. IA for the next 3x consecutive contractions).
- If concerns persist, start CTG.

Cardiotocogram/External Fetal Monitoring

- Do not offer cardiotocogram (CTG) to women at low risk of complications in established labour.
- Do not offer continuous CTG (cCTG) to women who have non-significant meconium if there are no other risk factors (**Table 5.5**).
- Do not regard amniotomy alone for suspected delay in the established first stage of labour as an indication to start cCTG.

TABLE 5.5

Indications for cCTG in Labour

Antenatal Risk Factors – cCTG Planned from Onset of Labour	
Maternal	• Maternal request • Medical co-morbidity – diabetes, hypertensive disorders including pre-eclampsia or cardiac, renal or thyroid condition
Labour related	• Prolonged spontaneous rupture of membranes (SROM) >24 hours
Iatrogenic	• VBAC or previous myomectomy • IOL
Fetal	• Gestation <37 or >42 • Abnormal Doppler artery velocimetry • Confirmed or suspected intrauterine growth restriction (IUGR) • Oligo or polyhydramnios • Malpresentation • Multiple pregnancy • Small for gestational age (SGA) or large for gestational age (LGA) • Reduced fetal movements (RFM) in past 24 hours • Two-vessel umbilical cord • Fetal structural abnormalities diagnosed antenatally and planned for continuous external fetal monitoring (cEFM)

(Continued)

TABLE 5.5 *(Continued)*

Indications for cCTG in Labour

Risk Factors Arising During Labour	
Maternal	• Maternal pulse over 120 beats/minute on two occasions 30 minutes apart • Temperature of 38°C or above on a single reading, or 37.5°C or above on two consecutive occasions 1 hour apart • *Severe hypertension*: a single reading of either systolic blood pressure of 160 mmHg or more or diastolic blood pressure of 110 mmHg or more, measured between contractions • *Hypertension*: either systolic blood pressure of 140 mmHg or more or diastolic blood pressure of 90 mmHg or more on 2 consecutive readings taken 30 minutes apart, measured between contractions • A reading of 2+ of protein on urinalysis and a single reading of either raised systolic blood pressure (140 mmHg or more) or raised diastolic blood pressure (90 mmHg or more)
Labour related	• Suspected chorioamnionitis or sepsis • Pain reported by the woman that differs from the pain normally associated with contractions • Presence of significant meconium • Fresh vaginal bleeding • Confirmed delay in the first or second stage of labour • Contractions that last longer than 60 seconds (hypertonus), or more than 5 contractions in 10 minutes (tachysystole)
Iatrogenic	• Oxytocin use • Epidural
Fetal	• Breech, oblique, transverse • Free floating head in primip • Recurrent accelerations (immediately following a contraction, i.e. overshoot) • Fetal heart rate (FHR) <110 or >160 or if FHR inappropriate for gestation • Rise in baseline FHR • 2x decelerations in FHR heard on (IA) after two successive contractions

6

Planned Birth in Special Circumstances

Preterm Birth

See **Tables 6.1** and **6.2**.

TABLE 6.1

Definitions

	Gestation
Term	37+0–41+6
Late preterm	32+0–36+6
Early preterm	29+0–31+6
Extremely preterm	22+0–27+6
Pre-viability	<= 21+6

TABLE 6.2

AN Risk Factors for Preterm Birth

Modifiable	• Smoking • Maternal age <18 yo • Domestic violence • <25 years old (yo) ⇑ risk for chlamydia and gonorrhoea	
Non-modifiable	*High risk**: ◀——— • Previous preterm birth (PTB) or mid trimester loss (16+0–34+0) • Previous cervical cerclage or progesterone • Trachelectomy • *Uterine variants*: septum, cornuate, intrauterine adhesions	These women will have had consultant-led care (CLC) with serial cervical length scanning 2–4 weekly between 14–24 weeks Cervical cerclage and progesterone reduce risk of PTB in women with risk factors + a short cervix
	Moderate risk*: ◀——— • Single LLETZ >15 mm depth excision • Multiple LLETZ ≤15 mm depth excision or cone biopsy	These women will have had CLC +/– a single cervical length scan at 18–22 weeks

* A term delivery since the event makes risk of PTB in current pregnancy lower.
Abbreviation: LLETZ, Large loop excision of the transformation zone

DOI: 10.1201/9781003508151-6

Diagnosis of Preterm Labour in Women with Intact Membranes

Assessment

Review of antenatal history

- Gestational age
- Review fetal growth surveillance
- Review risk factors for PTB

Preterm uterine contractions are common and don't always lead to PTB

Maternal assessment

History

- When did the contractions start?
- How often are the contractions?
- Are fetal movements felt?
- Has there been any vaginal loss? When? Colour?
- Preceding abdominal trauma?

Placental abruption?
Scar rupture?

Examination

Palpate Abdomen
- Assess contractions – for duration, strength and frequency.
- Does the uterus relax between contractions?
- Is there scar pain?
- Check for fetal lie, position and presentation and engagement.
- Consider bedside ultrasound scan (USS) to confirm presentation.

Speculum Examination
- Assess for bulging membranes.
- Assess for evidence of SROM.
- Assess for bleeding.
- Consider fetal fibronectin (FFN) or Actim Partus (depending on local guidelines, and if not able to perform cervical length assessment).
- Consider High vaginal swab (HVS) for microscopy, culture and sensitivity (MC+S).

Avoid lubricant if testing FFN

USS for fetal position and presentation
Transvaginal USS for cervical length is
the gold standard to diagnose PTL (if CL
<15mm).

Malposition is more common
in preterm babies

Investigations

- Urine dip to rule out UTI
- Full observations
- Full blood count (FBC), group and
  save (G+S), infection screen
- Cervical length scan

If history and investigations are suggestive of PTL, then follow management algorithm in **Figure 6.1**.

UTI?
PET
Chorioamnionitis?

Fetal Assessment

Cardiotocography (CTG) or auscultation
after contraction depending on gestation
(**Figures 6.1** and **6.2**).

Dawes Redman is contra-
indicated if there is uterine
activity

Mode of Delivery

Singleton Cephalic Baby

- Caesarean section (C/S) is not routinely recommended for a singleton
  cephalic baby.
- The process of vaginal birth may help initiate breathing and possibly reduce
  infections (including MRSA which is a cause of necrotising enterocolitis
  (NEC) in preterm babies).
- In a very preterm baby, a C/S may be indicated due to the risk of fetal dis-
  tress during labour. However, be aware of the following:
  - A very small baby can be difficult to deliver at C/S (particularly if trans-
    verse lie and/or reduced liquor volume).
  - The lower segment may be poorly formed necessitating a classical or
    upper segment C/S. This has ramifications for future deliveries.

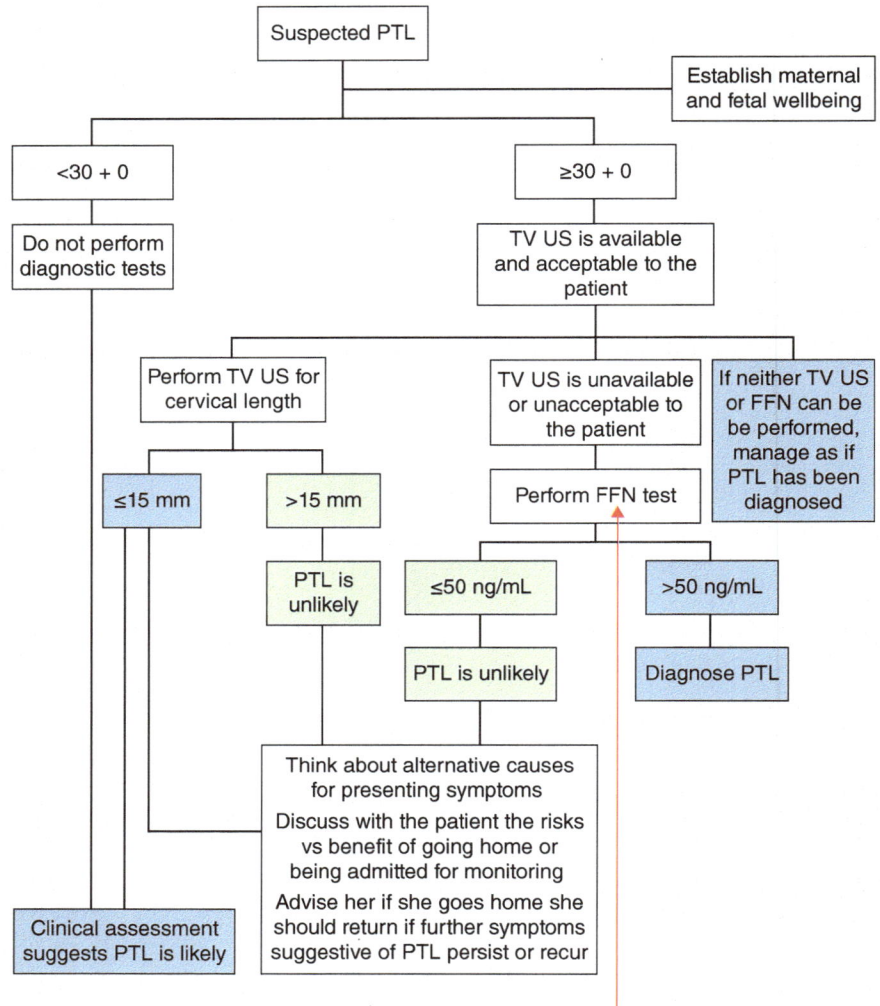

FIGURE 6.1   Management algorithm for suspected PTL.

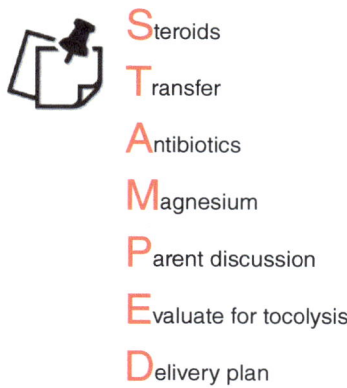

Steroids

Transfer

Antibiotics

Magnesium

Parent discussion

Evaluate for tocolysis

Delivery plan

FIGURE 6.2   Management plan.

Singleton Breech Baby

- Breech presentation is more common in preterm infants.
- Breech presentation is associated with increased incidence of neonatal mortality compared with cephalic preterm infants regardless of the mode of delivery
- Be vigilant for incomplete presentations such as footling breech. This is associated with cord prolapse.
- C/S is not routinely recommended for a singleton breech baby.
- The National Institute of Clinical Excellence (NICE; 2015) advises considering C/S for women presenting in suspected diagnosed or established preterm labour between 26+0 and 36+6 weeks of pregnancy with breech presentation.
- The Royal College of Obstetricians and Gynaecologists (RCOG; 2017) does not recommend routine C/S for breech presentation in spontaneous preterm labour at the threshold of viability 22–25+6.

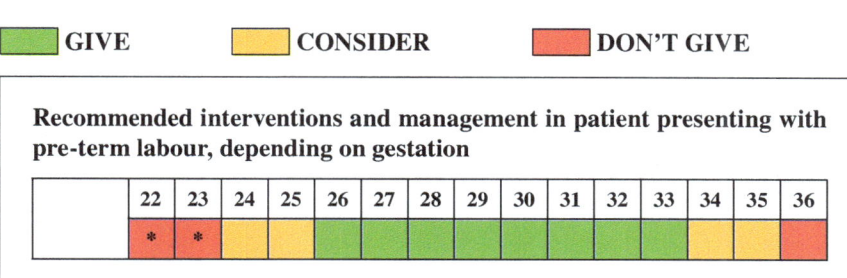

GIVE   CONSIDER   DON'T GIVE

Recommended interventions and management in patient presenting with pre-term labour, depending on gestation

	22	23	24	25	26	27	28	29	30	31	32	33	34	35	36
	*	*													

Regime
- Betamethasone 12 mg IM, two doses 24 hours apart
- Dexamethasone 6 mg IM, for four doses, 12 hours apart

Repeat courses
  • Consider in a select high risk group of women, considering the possible impact on fetal growth.
  • Consider a single repeat course of maternal corticosteroids for women less than 34+0 weeks of pregnancy who: have already had a course of corticosteroids when this was more than 7 days ago and are at very high risk of giving birth in the next 48 hours.

Cautions
  • Maternal side effects include pain at the injection site and, in diabetic women, a derangement in sugar control. Corticosteroids given in late preterm infants may also derange their sugars postnatally. Some evidence suggests steroids may be associated with an increase in cognitive and behavioural problems in childhood.

Magnesium sulphate

Gestation	22	23	24	25	26	27	28	29	30	31	32	33	34	35	36
	*	*													

Regime
  • *Loading dose*: 4 g magnesium sulphate over 15–20 minutes
  • *Maintenance dose*: 1 g/hour for up to 24 hours

This can be discontinued if the clinical situation changes, and imminent labour is subsequently thought unlikely.

Repeat courses
  • Avoid prolonged/repeated antenatal administration >5 days. Prolonged use is associated with neonatal skeletal adverse effects, hypocalcaemia and hypermagnesemia. However, repeat doses can be given if subsequently PTL appears likely again, and the benefits outweigh the risks. Discuss with the on-call consultant.

Cautions
  • Side effects (maternal)
    • Flushing
    • Sweating
    • Nausea and vomiting
    • Hypotension
    • Tachycardia
  • Polypharmacy
    • When given in conjunction with calcium channel antagonists (nifedipine), cardiovascular and neuromuscular effects may be exaggerated.

Toxicity
- Toxicity presents with muscle weakness and paralysis. It is unlikely at appropriate doses

Serum levels do not need to be checked (unless concerns about Mg toxicity) but monitoring for the duration of treatment is required as per local guidelines (at least 4 hourly).

Suggested monitoring
- Every 30 minutes
  - Respiratory rate
  - Pulse oximetry
- Every 4 hours
  - Blood pressure
  - Urine output
  - Tendon reflexes

Discontinue $MgSO_4$ if:

- Patellar reflexes are lost
- Urine output <30 mL/hour
- Respiratory rate <12/minute
- Weakness, nausea, sensation of warmth, flushing, drowsiness, double vision, and slurred speech

If magnesium sulphate toxicity is suspected, give calcium gluconate 1g IV

NB
- Delivery should not be delayed solely for magnesium sulphate administration.
- Magnesium sulphate infusions should not be used during antenatal transfer.

Tocoloysis

Gestation	22	23	24	25	26	27	28	29	30	31	32	33	34	35	36
	*	*													

Regime
- Nifedipine (First Line)
  - *Loading dose*: Oral nifedipine (immediate release) 10 mg on four occasions 20 minutes apart (i.e. 10 mg orally at 0, 20, 40 and 60 minutes) OR at 20-minute intervals until contractions stop, up to a maximum of four doses
  - *Maintenance dose*: Oral nifedipine modified release (MR) tablet 20 mg, given 4 hours after loading dose. This is followed by nifedipine MR 20 mg 8 hourly for 48 hours or until a decision is made to stop it.
- Atosiban (Second Line)
  - Atosiban is generally only used if nifedipine is contra-indicated (severe maternal cardiopulmonary compromise).

Cautions
- Side effects (maternal)
  - Nifedpine, especially immediate release, risks a sudden drop in blood pressure.
  - Monitoring for the duration of treatment is required as per local guidelines.
- Suggested regime during the loading dose
  - Maternal observations every 15 minutes
  - Continual CTG

Contra-indications to Tocolysis

- Ruptured membranes
- Advanced dilatation
- Significant APH
- Severe lethal anomaly
- Evidence of fetal compromise
- Evidence of maternal compromise (e.g. severe PET, sepsis)

NB
- There is no definitive evidence that tocolytics alter outcome.
- They are indicated to delay delivery for the administration of corticosteroids or to facilitate an in-utero transfer.

Antibiotic prophylaxis for group B streptococcus (GBS)

Gestation	22	23	24	25	26	26	28	29	30	31	32	33	34	35	36
	*	*													

Regime
- *Loading dose*: Benzylpenicillin 3 g IV bolus
- *Maintenance dose*: Benzylpenicillin 1.5 g IV 4 hourly until delivery

Cautions
- Penicillin allergy
  - Provided a woman has not had severe allergy to penicillin, a cephalosporin should be used.
  - If there is any evidence of severe allergy to penicillin, vancomycin should be used.

NB
- The risk of vertical transmission of GBS infection is higher in preterm infants and the mortality from neonatal GBS infection is higher than at term.

For women with known GBS colonisation with PPROM but no evidence of imminent PTL, the perinatal risks associated with PTB < 34+0 are likely to outweigh the risk of perinatal infection. Beyond 34+0 it may be beneficial to expedite delivery. Discuss with the on-call consultant obstetrician.

- Empirical intrapartum antibiotic prophylaxis against GBS should be given as soon as preterm labour is confirmed (or induced).
- Swabs for GBS are not recommended for women presenting with prelabour rupture of membranes (PPROM).
- GBS prophylaxis is not recommended for women with intact membranes having a planned preterm C/S.

In utero transfer to site with a NICU

Gestation	22	23	24	25	26	27	28	29	30	31	32	33	34	35	36
Singleton															
Multiples															
EFW <1500 g															

Contra-indications to in utero transfer (IUT)

- Active labour – if there is any doubt about the feasibility of IUT, the case should be discussed with the consultant obstetrician
- Maternal compromise
- Fetal compromise

Fetal monitoring

Gestation	22	23	24	25	26	27	28	29	30	31	32	33	34	35	36
Fetal scalp electrode (FSE)															
CTG/IA	*	*	*	*	*										

CTG/IA
- There is no evidence that CTG is better than intermittent auscultation (IA).
- NICE (2015) recommends that if prematurity is the only risk factor then either method is acceptable.
- Discuss with the on-call consultant obstetrician at gestations between 22+0–25+6.
- A Cochrane review (2017) found that continuous CTG in PTL increases the rates of instrument birth and C/S, that neonatal seizures were reduced but the rates of cerebral palsy were not.

- A normal CTG is reassuring, but a preterm CTG may be difficult to interpret:
  - They are likely to have an elevated baseline fetal heart rate (FHR) due to prematurity.
  - Decelerations may not be pathological.
  - Not all preterm babies with an abnormal CTG will be hypoxic or acidotic.
  - Loss of contact is more likely.

FSE
- Discuss with the patient the use of an FSE between 34+0–36+6 only if it has proven not possible to monitor the FHR via either CTG or IA.
- An FSE should be used with extreme caution <34+0.

To apply an FSE <34+0 ALL of the following must apply:

1. It is not possible to monitor the FHR via either CTG or IA.
2. The benefits are likely to outweigh the potential risks.
3. The alternatives (immediate birth or no monitoring) have been discussed with the woman and are unacceptable to her.
4. It has been discussed with a senior obstetrician.

ANALGESIA

Regional anaesthesia is not contra-indicated, though PTL may be quicker than a term delivery.
Avoid pethidine as it may cause neonatal respiratory depression, drowsiness and depressed reflexes, including feeding reflex, which is often poor anyway in a preterm baby.

OBSERVATIONS

Perform observations as per local policy for magnesium sulphate.
Women undergoing vaginal birth after caesarean (VBAC) should be closely monitored for features of scar rupture as usual.

AUGMENTATION

Due to the risk of cord prolapse, artificial rupture of membranes (ARM) is not recommended and there is also a risk of exacerbating ascending infection.
Oxytocin augmentation isn't contra-indicated, but a stalling in labour progress in a preterm delivery is likely to be desirable. Additionally, a preterm baby is more likely to be distressed by contractions. Only in a late preterm labour or where expedition of labour was solely for

maternal well-being (e.g. a very preterm baby and evidence of chorioamnionitis) would this be a consideration. This decision should be made by a consultant obstetrician.

FIRST STAGE

Prematurity is not an indication for routine C/S in established labour.
PTL is often faster than a term delivery, especially in a multip.
If the labour is considered high risk enough for gastric acid reducing agents to be given, be mindful that nifedipine for tocolysis will interact with cimetidine to cause hypotension (a proton pump inhibitor, e.g. omeprazole, should be first line).
There is no clear consensus on fetal monitoring in PTL (see above).
Preterm breech babies are more likely to present with incomplete presentations such as footling with associated risks of umbilical cord prolapse and a premature urge to push.

SECOND STAGE

Carry out expectant management.
If intervention is needed, be careful to touch only bony prominences of the fetus, and don't use excessive traction.

DELIVERY

Avoid fetal blood sampling (FBS) <34/40.
Avoid ventouse <34/40. If intervention at fully dilated is needed, forceps are favourable but may damage the skull. Intervention is less likely to be needed as the baby will be smaller.
Aim for delayed cord clamping, even if only 30 seconds is achievable (ideally 3 minutes), where possible. Be guided by the neonatologist.
Skin-to-skin contact improves clinical outcomes in late preterm babies, as with term babies.
Thermoregulation is important for preterm babies. Delivery into a plastic bag (without drying the baby first) may be advised by the neonatologist. This can be instigated prior to cord clamping.

THIRD STAGE

PTL does not increase risk of post-partum haemorrhage (PPH).
If the underlying cause of the PTL is PET, avoid ergometrine (this includes Syntometrine).
NICE (2015) recommends delayed cord clamping (DCC; **Table 6.3**) for 30 sec to 3 minutes for a well mother and preterm baby. It improves blood pressure during stabilization and reduces intraventricular haemorrhage, NEC and the need for blood transfusion (although jaundice requiring phototherapy is increased).
Anecdotally, retained placenta is more common with very early gestational births.

TABLE 6.3

Delayed Cord Clamping

Delayed cord clamping (DCC) for 30 sec to 3 minutes has been shown (NICE 2015) to	
☺ Improve blood pressure during fetal stabilisation ☺ Reduce the rate of intraventricular haemorrhage ☺ Reduce the rate of NEC ☺ Reduce the need for blood transfusion	☹ Increase the rates of jaundice requiring phototherapy

POSTPARTUM

Women should be routinely assessed for thromboprophylaxis as per local guidelines.

Counsel regarding the impact of PTL on subsequent pregnancy surveillance.

Management of Preterm Labour <26 Weeks' Gestation

- A senior neonatologist and a senior obstetrician should perform personalised counselling, using established predictors such as fetal gender and estimated fetal weight (EFW).
- The US National Institutes of Health Extremely Preterm Birth Outcomes Tool is freely available online (www.nichd.nih.gov/research/supported/EPBO).
- If time permits, a prior agreed management plan for the birth and resuscitation of the baby should be documented.
- Flexibility of plan is required as risk factors may change depending on fetal condition.

Counselling Elements

- The outlook including the predicted rates of mortality and morbidity by gestation
- Supportive care vs active resuscitation
  - In the absence of other complicating factors, there should be an expectation of resuscitation at 24+0 weeks and beyond
- Mode of delivery
- The benefits, risks and recommendations for interventions including
  - Corticosteroids
  - $MgSO_4$
  - Tocolytics
  - Intrapartum prophylactic antibiotics
  - Monitoring of the FHR in labour
  - Potential intrauterine transfer to a unit with a neonatal unit appropriate for the gestation

Mode of Delivery

- C/S is not routinely recommended for spontaneous PTL of either a cephalic or breech baby at the threshold of viability 22–25+6 (RCOG 2017).
- There are no known specific benefits or harms for the baby from delivery by C/S but the available evidence is very limited.
- Extracting a baby at the threshold of viability during a C/S can be difficult.
- The lower segment may not be well formed, necessitating a classical uterine incision. This has implications on future deliveries as a VBAC could not be recommended.
- A preterm baby may be small enough for fetal parts to descend through an incompletely dilated cervix. In the case of breech this includes entrapment of the aftercoming head or prolapse of the leg.

Fetal Monitoring

- There is limited evidence regarding the interpretation of CTGs in PTL.
- There is no evidence that a CTG improves the outcomes of preterm labour compared to IA.
- If monitoring is chosen, careful discussion and planning regarding how concerns arising from the monitoring would be managed should be had before they arise.
- If active resuscitation is planned at delivery it may stand to reason to monitor the baby in labour to inform resuscitation efforts.
- Not monitoring the FHR in labour is an option. This may be particularly appropriate <24/40 where a decision for supportive/comfort care only has been made.
- The choice to monitor an extremely preterm baby may not necessarily be because labour would be expedited in the event of distress; some parents may opt for monitoring to inform expectations of whether the baby will be alive at delivery.

Troubleshooting: A Patient presents with Threatened PTL but Contractions then Settle

There is no evidence that the following prevent further cervical dilatation and thus are not advised:

1. Total bed rest
2. Head-down positioning
3. Urinary catheter insertion

Contra-indications to rescue cerclage:

- Uterine contractions
- Significant vaginal bleeding/APH
- Ruptured membranes
- Evidence of chorioamnionitis
- Fetal parts prolapsed through the cervix

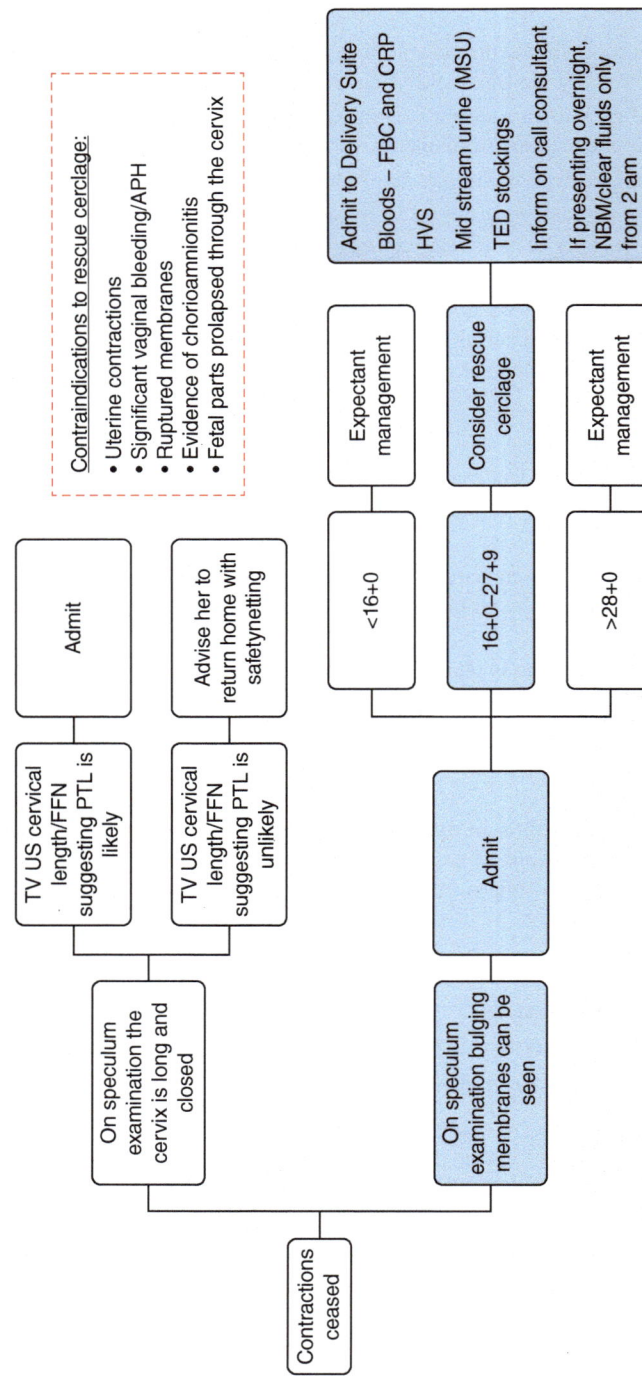

FIGURE 6.3   Algorithm that might lead to rescue cervical cerclage.

Rescue Cervical Cerclage

A rescue (or emergency) cervical cerclage describes a suture to draw the cervix into a closed position in an attempt to halt further dilatation. It may be appropriate (**Figures 6.3** and **6.4**) if a degree of cervical dilatation has occurred such that the membranes are exposed i.e. preterm prelabour bulging membranes. The aim is to prolong pregnancy and increase the gestational age at delivery, to avoid a 2nd trimester miscarriage or improve neonatal outcome. See **Figure 6.3** for clinical assessment which may lead to decision for rescue cervical cerclage.

Caution

- Rescue cerclage is performed only in specific circumstances to avoid iatrogenic morbidity.
- Progression of cervical dilatation is unpredictable, and every additional day in utero confers a survival benefit in extremely preterm babies. Inadvertent ROM may result in delivery, and potentially fetal demise, which may not have otherwise occurred.
- The short- and long-term risk vs benefit profile for rescue cerclage is largely unknown.
- If a patient with a cerclage in situ starts contracting regularly, it needs to be removed to avoid cervical trauma.

Complications of Rescue Cerclage

- Cervical trauma
- Infection/Sepsis
- Iatrogenic ROM and thus expedition of delivery

Table 6.4 shows a sample proforma for the documentation of PTL.

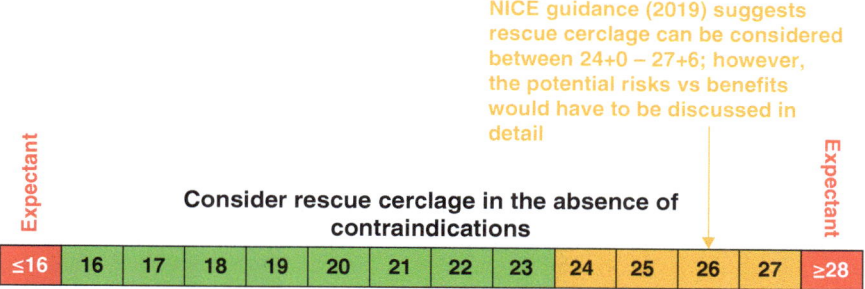

FIGURE 6.4 Gestations at which cervical cerclage should be offered or considered, and when to offer expectant management.

TABLE 6.4

Sample Proforma for Documentation of Preterm Labour

Gravida ____ Parity ____
Current gestational age: ____ weeks ____ days
Singleton/multiple pregnancy (and chorionicity): ____

Previous obstetric history: ____

Most recent ultrasound scan: ____ Date: ____
EFW: ____
Fetal sex: ____

Admission monitoring (CTG/IA): ____

Contractions: ____/10
Cervical dilation: ____ cm

Membranes
• Intact
• Ruptured
  Date: ____ Time: ____

Presentation on bedside ultrasound: ____

Maternal/Fetal risk factors
☐ Maternal infection/chorioamnionitis
☐ GBS positive
☐ Maternal diabetes/hypertension
☐ Antepartum haemorrhage
☐ Abnormal anomaly scan/screening
☐ Intrauterine growth restriction (IUGR) and/or abnormal Dopplers

Interventions

* Corticosteroids
[1] Date: ____ Time: ____
[2] Date: ____ Time: ____

• Magnesium sulphate
[Loading] Date: ____ Time: ____
[Maintenance] Date: ____ Time: ____

• Tocoloysis
[Loading] Date: ____ Time: ____
[Maintenance] Date: ____ Time: ____

• Abx
[Loading] Date: ____ Time: ____
[Maintenance] Date: ____ Time: ____

Plans

Fetal monitoring
☐ No monitoring of FH
☐ Intermittent auscultation
☐ Continuous CTG

Level of management agreed with parents and neonatologist:

☐ Active (survival focussed)
☐ Passive (comfort focussed)

VBAC

Quick check for a women presenting in labour with a history of prior C/S

☐ *Assessment of labour progression*: is she in active labour (if so admit to CLU). If not in established labour (NIEL) but contracting, consider admission for monitoring CTG if regular tightenings.

☐ *Suspicion of scar rupture*: If there are concerns about scar dehiscence or rupture at presentation, consider expedition of delivery via C/S.

☐ *Assessment of fetal wellbeing*: If there are concerns about fetal wellbeing at presentation consider expedition of delivery via C/S.

☐ *Placental site on prior ultrasound scans*: (There is increased risk of placenta praevia and invasive placenta if prior C/S.

☐ *Contra-indications to VBAC*
  • Prior classical C/S
  • Prior uterine rupture
  • Prior myomectomy breaching the myometrium

☐ *Special circumstances*
  • Multiple prior C/S
  • Preterm
  • Postdates
  • Twins
  • Advanced maternal age
  • Suspected macrosomia
  • Antenatal (AN) stillbirth (SB)

Counsel patient for mode of delivery following previous C/S using the statistics in **Figure 6.5**.

Assessment

Review of antenatal history

  • Gestational age
  • Review fetal growth surveillance
  • Review placental site
  • Review prior delivery/op notes

Ensure the prior uterine incision doesn't necessitate ERCS

Ensure the placenta is not low lying

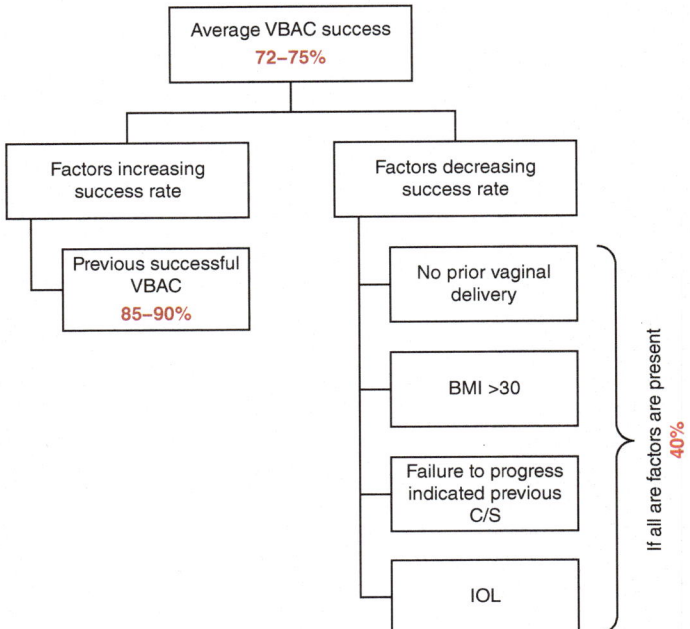

FIGURE 6.5   Factors in VBAC success.

Maternal assessment

History

- When did the contractions start?
- How often are the contractions?
- Are fetal movements felt?
- Has there been any vaginal loss? When? Colour?

Examination

Palpate Abdomen

- Assess contractions for duration, strength and frequency.
- Does the uterus relax between contractions?
- Is there scar pain?
- For fetal lie, position and presentation and engagement.
- Consider bedside USS to confirm presentation.

Vaginal Examination

- Cervical dilation
- Is there per vaginal (PV) bleeding?

Investigations

- FBC + G+S
- Full observation

Fetal Assessment

- CTG

Plan

- CLU with neonatal team access
- IV access
- Regular observations
- Continuous external fetal monitoring (cEFM)
- 1-to-1 care
- Careful monitoring of progression to identify labour dystocia, scar rupture or maternal/fetal compromise
- No less than 4-hourly assessment of dilatation from 4 cm
- Epidural not contra-indicated (though note increased requirement for pain relief may suggest rupture)
- Obstetric review if concerns re progression – careful consideration re augmentation of a VBAC

Uterine Rupture

See **Table 6.5**.

TABLE 6.5

The Risk of Uterine Rupture

Elective repeat caesarean section (ERCS)	0.02% (2 per 10,000)
Spontaneous onset VBAC	0.2–0.5% (20–50 per 10,000)

Presentation

The clinical features associated with uterine scar rupture include

- Abnormal CTG – the most consistent finding but not always present
- Severe abdominal pain, especially if persisting between contractions
- Acute onset scar tenderness
- Abnormal vaginal bleeding
- Haematuria
- Cessation of previously efficient uterine activity

- Maternal tachycardia, hypotension, fainting or shock
- Loss of station of the presenting part
- Change in abdominal contour and inability to pick up fetal heart rate at the old transducer site

Factors Increasing Uterine Rupture Risk

- Previous uterine rupture (>/= 5% recurrence risk) (VBAC contra-indicated)
- Previous classical C/S (VBAC contra-indicated)
- Insufficient evidence for J, T, low vertical uterine extensions (VBAC contra-indicated)
- Myomectomy at least equivalent to VBAC case-by-case + senior decision
- Short inter-delivery interval (<12 months since last delivery)
- Post-dates pregnancy
- Maternal age ≥40 years or more
- Obesity (particularly if BMI >40)
- Lower prelabour Bishop score
- Macrosomia
- Decreased ultrasonographic lower segment myometrial thickness.

VBAC in Special Circumstances

VBAC IOL/Augmentation

- VBAC induction of labour (IOL)/augmentation is associated with a 2–3x increased risk of uterine rupture and a 1.5x increased risk of Em C/S.
- IOL using mechanical methods is associated with a lower risk of uterine rupture (NICE 2021)
  - 8/1,000 for IOL with mechanical agent
  - 24/1,000 with prostaglandins (contra-indicated in a VBAC)
- Senior obstetric review is required to sanction a VBAC IOL and clear documentation of examination intervals and when to take recourse to C/S should be made.
- It is helpful to print off your local VBAC guidance and put it in the women's labour notes as it is likely to have a flow chart for frequency of examinations and when to diagnose delay for ease of reference.
- IOL/augmentation should occur on labour ward with access to continual fetal monitoring and immediate access to C/S.

≥2 Previous C/S

- VBAC success rate is 71.1%.
- Uterine rupture rate is 1.36%.
- The maternal morbidity associated with a VBAC is comparable to an ERCS.

- The maternal morbidity associated with a VBAC following 2x previous C/S is higher compared to a VBAC following 1x previous C/S:
  - Hysterectomy (56/10,000 compared with 19/10,000)
  - Transfusion (1.99% compared with 1.21%)
- Following a comprehensive individualised risk assessment by a senior obstetrician, a fully informed women's wish to have a VBAC can be supported.

≥41+0 Weeks of Gestation

- NICE (2021) recommends induction of labour from 41+0 in general. It makes no specific mention of VBAC delivery. In general, IOL at 41+0 reduces perinatal mortality without an increase in caesarean delivery rates.
- The risk of stillbirth ≥ 39 weeks is two-fold higher in women with a previous C/S (11 per 10,000 or 0.11%) compared with women without previous C/S (5 per 10,000 or 0.05%) (absolute risks 11 per 10,000.
- Therefore, the reduction in risk of SB that occurs by delivering from 41 weeks is likely to be greater among women with a previous C/S. However, this must be balanced against the risks of VBAC IOL compared with spontaneous VBAC labour: 2–3x increased risk of uterine rupture and 1.5x increased risk of emergency C/S.
- It is not unreasonable therefore in a woman who would elect for a VBAC were labour to spontaneously start but who would not want a VBAC IOL, to schedule a provisional ERCS at around 41 weeks and await events.

Maternal age ≥40 Years

- Maternal age ≥40 years is an independent risk factor for SB.
- Previous C/S is an independent risk factor for SB.
- Maternal age ≥40 years is an independent risk factor for unsuccessful VBAC.
- There is insufficient evidence to guide timing of delivery in women ≥40 yo who have previously had a C/S but desire a VBAC.
- In general, evidence suggests consideration of delivery by 39+0–40+0 to avoid the SB risk; however, this needs to be balanced against the risks of VBAC IOL compared with spontaneous VBAC labour.

Preterm VBAC

- Planned VBAC success rates for preterm and term pregnancies are similar.
- Perinatal outcomes are similar with preterm VBAC and preterm ERCS.
- The rates of uterine rupture are lower for preterm VBAC compared to term VBAC (34 per 10,000 vs 74 per 10,000).

Twins

- There is no definitive evidence nor guidance in twin VBAC deliveries to inform counselling. As such, caution is advised if a VBAC is being considered in a multiple pregnancy.

Suspected Fetal Macrosomia

- EFW ≥4 kg is associated with an increased risk of
  - Uterine rupture
  - Unsuccessful VBAC
  - Shoulder dystocia
  - Obstetric anal sphincter injury (OASI)
- Studies suggest the likelihood of a successful VBAC of a macrosomia baby in a woman without prior successful vaginal delivery is <50%.
- However, 3rd trimester ultrasound is a poor predictor of fetal size.

IUD

- Women with an antepartum fetal demise have an 87% success rate for VBAC delivery; however, as deliveries of an intrauterine death (IUD) often required IOL, the risk of uterine rupture remains. Consider how to monitor for this in the absence of FHR abnormalities as a sign.

Breech

Figure 6.6 demonstrates the types of breech presentation and risk of cord prolapse.

> Frank/extended breech likely to have a successful vaginal delivery than other positions as the bottom makes a good fit so cold prolapse is less likely and feet/knees are less likely to obstruct.

> Footling breech – higher risk of cord prolapse and complications

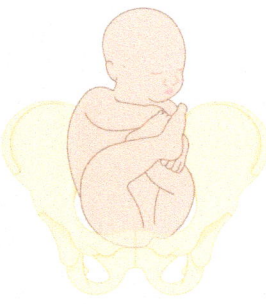
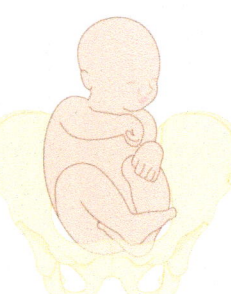
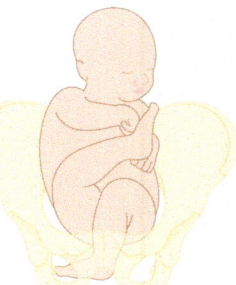

FRANK BREECH   COMPLETE BREECH   FOOTLING BREECH

FIGURE 6.6 Types of breech.

Breech Presenting in Labour

- There is no evidence to support Em C/S for a labouring breech.
- IOL is not usually recommended in breech.
- A multip who has had a previous vaginal birth is less likely to have complications with a vaginal breech delivery.
- Keep the baby sacroanterior to deliver. If the back is facing the wrong way (sacroposterior) then term breech birth is unlikely, and a C/S will be indicated.
- Hands off the delivering breech!

See **Table 6.6** for a summary of counselling points.

TABLE 6.6

Quick Counselling

In Favour of		Caveats
Vaginal birth	Successful vaginal breech carries lower maternal complications than elective caesarean section (El C/S)	But the highest risk category is emergency caesarean section (Em C/S) (40% of vaginal breech → Em C/S)
	C/S increases the risk in future pregnancies: 1. Abnormally invasive placenta 2. Complications of repeat C/S 3. Small increased risk of SB	
El C/S	Planned vaginal breech birth increases the risk of low Apgar scores and serious short-term complications	But has not been shown to increase the risk of long-term morbidity
	El LSCS leads to a small reduction in perinatal mortality compared to planned vaginal breech delivery	This is due to three factors, only one of which is unique to breech: 1. Avoidance of SB after 39 weeks of gestation 2. Avoidance of intrapartum risks 3. Avoidance of risks of vaginal breech delivery.

Approach to Initial Assessment of Patient Presenting in Labour with Breech Presentation

1. **Assess fetal well-being**	⇒	Signs of fetal distress (FD)	⇒ C/S if not FD
2. **Vaginal examination**	⇒	Cord prolapse	⇒ C/S if not FD
	⇒	Footling breech	C/S if not FD
3. **Review AN history**	⇒	Twins	⇒ Routine C/S is recommended if the leading twin is breech Routine C/S is not recommended if the second twin is breech (as long as first is cephalic)
	⇒	Preterm	⇒ Routine C/S is not recommended unless it is planned due to maternal or fetal compromise Routine C/S at the threshold of viability (22–22+6) is not recommended
	⇒	VBAC?	⇒ Consider C/S
4. **Review ultrasound (US) scans**	⇒	LGA	⇒ Consider C/S
	⇒	SGA	⇒ Consider C/S
5. **Perform bedside US**	⇒	Hyperextended neck	⇒ Consider C/S

Latent phase of labour	
There may be a long latent phase due to a lack of application of presenting part to cervix.	
First stage of labour	
Location	CLU
Analgesia	Women should have a choice of analgesia. Routine epidural is not advised. Epidural may increase intervention (RCOG 2017).
Contractions	The woman may feel breathless during or after contractions due to the pressure of the baby's head on her diaphragm. She may experience the pain more in her back than the front.
Maternal position	Women should be encouraged to adopt whatever position feels best. The PROMPT manual (2012) states that women should be routinely advised to assume lithotomy position for birth since this is what most staff experienced in breech birth are used to.
Fetal presentation	The presenting part is often higher in the pelvis than a cephalic presentation and the station is likely to go up and down more during labour.
Fetal monitoring	Following spontaneous rupture of membranes (SROM), perform a vaginal examination (VE) to exclude cord prolapse and check fetal heart for any effects of cord compression. RCOG (2017) states that continuous electronic fetal monitoring should be offered to women with a breech in labour. PROMPT (2012) suggests an FSE may be placed on baby bottom but FSE on bottom may risk injury particularly to scrotum.
Delay?	Avoid routine ARM. Augmentation of labour is not advised unless slow progress.
Second stage	
Passive:	RCOG (2017) recommends passive second stage of an hour to allow the breech to descend.
Active:	Hands off approach and intervene only if needed. RCOG (2017) does not recommend routine assisted breech delivery over spontaneous birth Frank meconium is to be expected due to pressure on the baby as it descends through the birth canal. Some suggest membranes should be broken when the buttocks reach the perineum to allow any meconium to drain from the vagina. However, the membranes usually break spontaneously as the legs are born. Meconium does not necessarily suggest stress; however, meconium-stained liquor in labour should be assessed and responded to in the same way as for a cephalic delivery.
The birth	
When handling baby, hold only bony prominences (thumbs on sacrum and fingers on hip bones; PROMPT 2012). Do not pull: Forceful traction by the deliverer may cause iatrogenic brain and spinal injuries, nuchal arm, hyperextended head.	

Management of a Vaginal Breech Delivery, and Troubleshooting for Potential Complications

Complications		Interventions
Umbilical cord prolapse	Manage as per cephalic presentation cord prolapse. If the cervix is fully dilated vaginal birth may still be possible particularly for multips or if baby is not large It is more common if preterm, footling, second twin, or after ARM.	
Delay?	RCOG (2017) recommends C/S for breech if not visible within 2 hours of active pushing.	
Presenting part	A rocking or up and down motion during descent of the baby's bottom ('rumping') is the equivalent of 'crowning' in a cephalic birth.	
Buttocks	The buttocks are born by lateral flexion.	
		RCOG (2017) does not advocate routine episiotomy in breech birth. Perform episiotomy when bottom is at the perineum to expedite birth if fetal compromise.
Delay?	RCOG (2017) defines slow progress as a delay of more than 5 minutes from delivery of the buttocks to the head or of more than 3 minutes from the umbilicus to the head.	
Shoulders	Simultaneously body rotates so that the shoulders drop into the transverse diameter of the pelvic brim (the widest diameter).	
		If delay, perform Løvsett's manoeuvre.
Arms	The arms will be born with spontaneous rotation of the baby.	
Nuchal arm	Traction on fetal trunk or legs risks a nuchal arm. Nuchal arms can be released using Løvsett's manoeuvre and running your hand along the fetal arm to the antecubital fossa and applying pressure to flex the arm	
Cord compression	As the arms are born the cord may be compressing against the baby's head and maternal pelvis. Wharton's jelly affords some protection but expect fetal heart rate to be slower. There is no evidence of any benefit in bringing down a little cord to relieve tension; this may in fact tighten a nuchal cord or cause the cord to go into spasm (PROMPT 2012)	
Trunk		Ensure baby remains sacro-anterior. If trunk is rotating to sacro-posterior, gently rotate back.
Delay?	RCOG (2017) defines slow progress as a delay of more than 3 minutes from the umbilicus to the head.	
Legs	The legs are released by the baby extending the pelvis around the maternal symphysis pubis.	
		The legs may need to be released by applying pressure to the popliteal fossae.

Head		Further rotation occurs so the head and the pelvis in the same diameter as if it were cephalic. The baby makes a tummy scrunch movement – flexing its legs up towards abdomen and scrunching shoulders as if trying to do a sit up – to facilitate head flexion. Internal head restitution occurs in a similar way to a cephalic birth.
		If delay: Bracht manoeuvre, Mauriceau-Smellie-Veit (MSV) manoeuvre or forceps delivery of the aftercoming head. If manoeuvres and forceps have failed→ symphysiotomy or LSCS
	Head entrapment	The average diameter of a term baby's bottom (bi-trochanteric) is 9 cm, and its head diameter (bi-parietal) is 9.5 cm. Therefore, head entrapment at term is unlikely as bottom has already delivered. If the baby is preterm, its head is often larger than its bottom, so head entrapment is more likely. Head entrapment is more likely if maternal pushing occurs prior to full dilation, as the legs and body may be born through cervix that is less than 10cm dilated, but the fetal head will not fit. If cervical incision is required to release an entrapped head, incise cervix at 10 and 2 o'clock to avoid the cervical neurovascular bundles. Be aware these can extend into the lower segment of the uterus.
Third stage		
Give oxytocin once birth of the baby's head is completed		
	Premature placental separation	It is thought – especially in standing positions in labour – that the centre of gravity is higher in a breech than cephalic birth, resulting in more traction being placed on the cord and placenta by gravity.

Deflection and Hyperextension (Stargazing) of the Baby's Head

- A deflection of the head and hyperextension can occur antenatally due to fetal or uterine abnormalities, placental location or a nuchal cord.
- Deflection may also occur in labour often resolving spontaneously.
- It may have persisted from antenatally or occur during birth itself.
- It can also be caused by unnecessary interventions such as traction on the legs causing extension of the head and arms.
- Assistance may be used to flex the head (e.g. MSV manoeuvre).
- Hyperextension – i.e. more extreme deflection – is often diagnosed by ultrasound.
- If detected at term, a C/S is usually advised.

Manoeuvres

Bracht Manoeuvre

Following spontaneous delivery to the level of the umbilicus, grasp the body with both hands, keeping legs flexed against abdomen. Without traction bring the body up against the symphysis pubis accompanied with suprapubic pressure.

(This is an alternative for the Burns-Marshall technique which RCOG 2017 discourages as it risks deflexing the head. The Burns-Marshall technique is allowing baby to hang to encourage descent; when the nape of the neck is visible, grasp the baby's ankles and tilt the body in an arc over the mother's abdomen.)

Do not assist flexion, by inserting finger in baby's mouth as traction on the jaw may cause dislocation.

Mauriceau–Smellie–Veit Manoeuvre

- Straddle the baby on your non-dominant forearm.
- Place two fingers of your non-dominant hand on the baby's cheek bones. (Do not put in baby's mouth.)
- With your dominant hand, place your outermost fingers on each side of the baby's shoulders and your middle finger on the occiput.
- Flex the baby's head.

Løvsett's Manoeuvre

- Grasp baby with thumbs over the sacrum and fingers on hips.
- Rotate the baby so one shoulder is anterior.
- Put index finger on shoulder and follow arm to antecubital fossa.
- Flex the anterior arm for delivery.
- Rotate baby 180 degrees keeping the back uppermost.
- Deliver the second arm in the same way as the first.

Forceps Delivery of the Aftercoming Head

- Assistant holds the baby.
- Apply forceps underneath the baby's body. (Apply in the same way as for a cephalic presentation, ensuring that the curve of the forceps follows the pelvic curve.)
- Axis of traction aims to flex the head.

Total Breech Extraction

- This is when a baby is extracted by the feet down through the birth canal.
- It risks head entrapment and nuchal arms.
- It is usually considered only for a non-cephalic second twin (and often follows an IPV when the operator has hold of the baby's feet).

Planned Twin Delivery

See **Figures 6.7** and **6.8**.

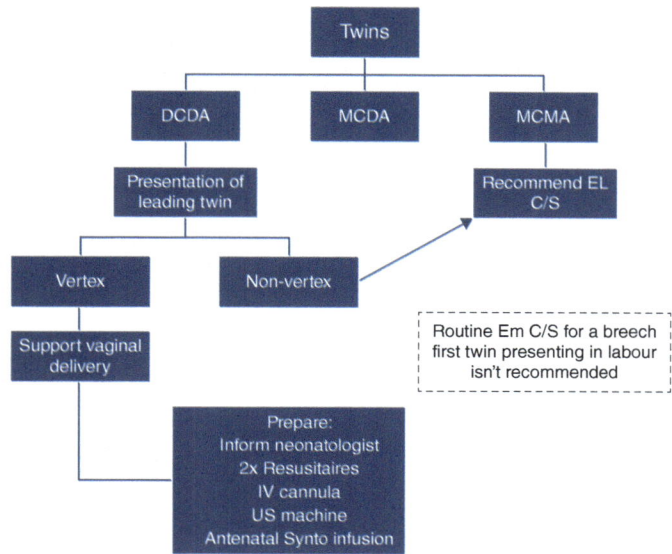

FIGURE 6.7 Deciding mode of delivery in twin pregnancies. *Abbreviations*: DCDA, dichorionic diamniotic; MCDA, monochorionic, diamniotic; MCMA, monochorionic, monoamniotic.

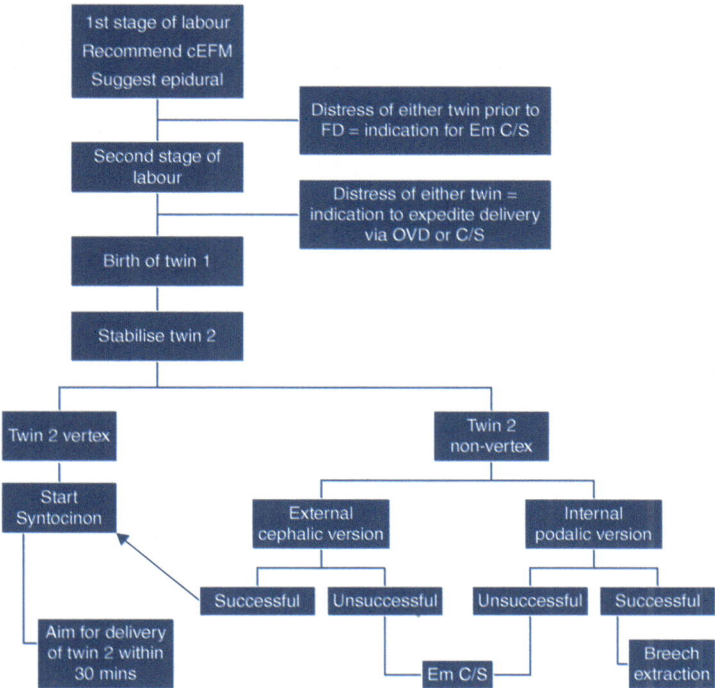

FIGURE 6.8 Management of labour in a twin pregnancy.

Intrapartum care for a twin pregnancy
• cCTG is recommended.   • Ensure that you offset the fetal heart beats on the CTG machine settings to avoid inadvertently monitoring the same baby twice   • If loss of contact of the abdominal transducer is encountered, a low threshold to apply an FSE to the scalp of the leading twin is advised.

Second stage of labour		
Delivery of twin 1	• Second-stage management for the delivery of the first twin should be carried out as per singleton deliveries.	
Inter-twin delivery time	**Management of Twin 1**	**Management of Twin 2**
	• Delayed cord clamping is the gold standard for most deliveries. • However, consider the chorionicity of twins – it is advised in monochorionic twins that the cord is cut is cut shortly after the birth of twin 1 due to theoretical concerns of twin-to-twin transfusion syndrome. • Skin-to-skin is the gold standard for most deliveries. • However, the mother may be distracted by the next delivery, so skin-to-skin with the partner may be more appropriate.	• The interval between the birth of the twin 1 and the birth of twin 2 is the time where complications are most likely to arise. • Transabdominal stabilisation of the fetal lie of twin 2 is important. Hold the baby in a longitudinal axis until the presenting part descends into the pelvis. • Avoid routine ARM (risk of cord prolapse). • In the absence of CTG concerns, allow 30 minutes between deliveries. • Do not assume that twin 2 is of a similar size to twin 1
Delivery of twin 2	• *Start a timer*: in the absence of concerns, 30 minutes can be allowed between deliveries before intervention is required. • There may be a gap in contractions. • Routine ARM is not advised due to the risk of cord prolapse (especially when the head is not engaged in the pelvis). • Syntocinon can be given (but only if the lie is longitudinal). • As contractions resume, the presenting part begins to descend into the pelvis. • Stabilise fetal lie until the presenting part descends. • A VE +/– US scan is appropriate at this stage to ascertain lie and presentation. • CTG changes are to be anticipated: • A prolonged deceleration or bradycardia should raise suspicion of a malposition or cord prolapse.	
	? What if twin 2 is breech? Deliver the baby breech or perform external cephalic version.	**? What if twin 2 is transverse?** Perform internal podalic version (turning a transverse lie to breech) or if this not possible expedite delivery by Em C/S.

Third stage of labour
• Active management is advised due to the increased PPH risk including third stage infusion of 40 iu of oxytocin   • Clamp cords in a way you can remember which is which – one clamp for baby one and two for baby two.   • Paired umbilical cord gases per baby are required.   • Deliver both twin placentas together by controlled cord traction as per singletons.

Body Mass Index >40 in Labour

For additional antenatal assessments, see **Figure. 6.9**.

BMI > 30	BMI > 35	BMI > 40
VTE risk assessment HTN/PET risk assessment GDM screening 5 mg folic acid Advise Vit D	As per BMI >30, plus Serial scans Consider aspirin from 12 weeks	As per BMI >35, plus Anaesthetic review 3rd trimester moving and handling assessment 3rd trimester assessment for tissue viability issues and planning Consider reweighing in 3rd trimester to make appropriate plans

FIGURE 6.9 Additional antenatal assessments.

Delivery Planning

AN plan for labour should made by 36/40 and documented in notes.

Mode of Delivery

- There are no specific guidelines recommending one form of delivery over another.
- Obesity is not an indication for routine El C/S.
- The decision to have an elective C/S indicated solely for obesity requires a multi-disciplinary team (MDT) decision and should be discussed with each woman on an individual basis.

Planned Vaginal Delivery

- *Location*: CLU advised
- Availability of senior obstetrician and anaesthetist.
- Absence of guidance recommending any amendments to analgesia and anaesthesia availability:
  - Anticipate a potentially difficult regional anaesthesia siting. (Therefore, early siting of an epidural is often preferred.)
  - Be mindful of moving and handling difficulties if there is maternal or fetal distress whilst in water.
- *Intrapartum fetal monitoring*: There is no specific guidance; therefore, act in accordance with standard NICE guidance for indications for cCTG. Loss of contact is more likely and early recourse to apply an FSE should be considered.

Elective C/S

- Obesity is associated with an increased risk of labour complications and an Em C/S (especially in advanced labour) is likely to be more challenging than an El C/S.

- NICE recommends that to reduce wound infection and separation rates a patient with >2 cm of subcutaneous fat should have the layer sutured.
- There is inadequate evidence to support any other specific surgical techniques in the setting of obesity, but suggested alterations may include the following:
  - Prophylactic antibiotics may be administered due to the increased risk of wound infection.
  - There is inadequate evidence for the routine use of negative pressure dressings, but local policies may vary.
  - There is inadequate evidence for the routine use of subcutaneous drains.
  - A retractor such as the 'Alexis O' may be helpful for access and visualisation of the surgical field.
  - Consider a slower-dissolving suture (e.g. loop PDS) to close the rectus sheath to reduce the risk of hernia formation.

Timing of Delivery

- There are no specific guidelines for the timing of delivery in obesity.
- SB risk is known to be increased.
- IOL at term may reduce the chance of C/S without increasing adverse outcomes. This should be discussed with each woman on an individual basis.

Delivery in Special Circumstances

- *Macrosomia*: Offer IOL as per usual macrosomia guidance.
- *Post-dates*: No specific guidance but increased risk of SB in obese women.
- *VBAC*: BMI > 30 carries a higher rate of failed VBAC. Implement an individualised counselling and plan.

Table 6.7 shows the documentation required on admission in labour for patients with raised BMI.

Plan

Immediate

1. Admit to CLU.
2. Inform on-call anaesthetist.
3. Inform on-call obstetrician.
4. Inform theatre team to ensure bariatric theatre bed availability.
5. Ensure availability of bariatric equipment on LW.
6. Review AN plan for labour.
7. Review moving and handling assessment.
8. Secure early venous access + consider 2nd cannula.
9. Ensure bloods up to date and group and save valid. Repeat if not.
10. Perform bedside scan to establish presentation if unclear from abdominal palpation.

TABLE 6.7

Documentation on Admission in Labour

Maternal age: ....

Maternal BMI: ....
Parity: ....
Gestational age: ....

Review of AN notes:
Maternal co-morbidities:
- Gestational diabetes mellitus (GDM)
- Hypertension (HTN)
- Pre-eclamptic toxaemia (PET)

AN VTE assessment:
RCOG score: ....
- Low-molecular-weight heparin (LMWH)
- Heparin
- No anticoagulation

If anticoagulated:
Last dose received: ....

Fetal AN assessment:
Screening results: ....

Growth surveillance:
- small for gestational age (SGA)
- large for gestational age (LGA)

First Stage of Labour

1. Continuous midwifery care in established labour
2. Vigilance for tissue viability issues; regular rolling if regional analgesia used
3. Early request for regional analgesia if desired due to possible difficulty siting
4. Assessment of need for continuous fetal monitoring; low threshold for FSE if unable to monitor well
5. Discuss with anaesthetist regarding appropriateness of eating and drinking, and need for PPI prophylaxis
6. Routine monitoring of labour progression unless concerns

Second Stage of Labour

1. Low threshold to suspect shoulder dystocia

Third Stage of Labour

1. Anticipate PPH
2. Active management of the 3rd stage

Intrapartum Care of Women at Known Risk of Bleeding

See **Table 6.8**.

TABLE 6.8

Antenatal Risk Factors and Care Implications

ANTENATAL RISK FACTORS	
Placenta praevia/accreta	• Placenta accreta likely to have planned delivery in specialist accreta centre • Presence of consultant obstetrician and anaesthetist • Blood products • Consent to include hysterectomy in event of massive PPH • Prophylactic vascular catheter placement (interventional radiology [IR]) to be considered • Consultant obstetrician planned and directly supervising delivery • Local availability of a level 2 critical care bed • Cell salvage if blood products not accepted
Bleeding/Clotting disorder	See sections on gestational thrombocytopenia, haemophilia and von Willebrand's disease (VWD)
Placental abruption – significant	• Significant antepartum haemorrhage (APH) is an indication for IOL if gestation is appropriate. The aim of IOL is to deliver the baby before a potential further or more significant bleed occurs. • APH is a risk factor for PPH; therefore, active management of the third stage as a minimum is advised. • The management of major APH is covered in Chapter 9
Multiple pregnancy	• Consultant-led unit (CLU) delivery
Hb <85	• Treat anaemia antenatally
Grandmultip	• Cannula in situ
Baby > 4 kg	• Active management of 3rd stage:
IUD	• *Vaginal delivery*: ergometrine–oxytocin (Syntometrine 500 µg/5 units) intramuscular (IM) in the absence of HTN
PET	• *C/S*: oxytocin (5 units by slow IV injection)
Previous PPH	• + Oxytocin infusion (40 units over 4 hours)
BMI >40	• Consider tranexamic acid (TXA) 1g IV
Uterine fibroids	• Consider XM 2-4units of RBC prior to delivery
Recurrent APH (minor)	
INTRAPARTUM RISK FACTORS	
Induction/augmentation of labour	
Sepsis/Pyrexia in labour	
Prolonged active 1st stage	
Prolonged syntocinon use	
Prolonged 2nd stage	
Em C/S	
Operative vaginal delivery (OVD)	

Idiopathic Thrombocytopenia (ITP) and Gestational Thrombocytopenia

See **Table 6.9**.

TABLE 6.9

Management of Thrombocytopenia in Pregnancy, Labour and Postnatally

Antenatal	Monitor maternal platelets at least weekly from 36/40.
Peripartum	If platelet count <50, discuss a delivery plan with MDT including haematologist. Consider steroids or IVIg to increase platelet count.
Intrapartum	Regional anaesthesia is contra-indicated if platelets <50 × 10^9/L (50–80 × 10^9/L = individualised decision). *Gestational thrombocytopenia (GT)*: Assume the baby does not have an increased bleeding risk. *ITP*: Assume the baby will be at increased risk of bleeding irrespective of maternal platelet count; therefore: Avoid • FBS • Ventouse Caution with • FSE • Midcavity or rotational forceps
Postpartum	• Perform active management of the 3rd stage with routine tranexamic acid. • IV immunoglobulin and/or steroids may be needed. • Avoid PN non-steroidal anti-inflammatory drugs (NSAIDs) and IM injections. • Postpartum follow with a haematologist +/− tapering of steroids. • Standard postpartum thromboprophylaxis risk assessment should be performed. If it is indicated LMWH can be given 6 hours post-delivery if lochia is normal + no evidence of bleeding elsewhere + platelet count of >50 × 10^9/L. ITP: Cord blood will be obtained to analyse the cord blood platelet count to inform fetal management.

Haemophilia

See **Table 6.10** and **Figure 6.10**.

TABLE 6.10

Management of Haemophilia in Pregnancy, Labour and Postnatally

Antenatal	Delivery plan to be made by 37/40.	
Peripartum	Clotting factors should be given as close to delivery as possible. Check plasma clotting factors before and after infusion, and at 4–6 hours following treatments. Desmopressin (DDAVP) has antidiuretic effects; therefore, restrict fluid to 1L/24hours to avoid hyponatraemia.	
Intrapartum	Regional anaesthesia requires factor VIII/IX levels of >0.5 iu/mL. Avoid IM injections if VIII/IX levels of <0.5 iu/mL. Female carriers are at increased risk of bleeding – the labouring mother or a female neonate. Male neonates are at risk of iatrogenic bleeding following delivery (e.g. intracranial haemorrhage). If status of baby unknown, treat as if affected.	In affected male and severely affected female neonates, avoid • ECV • FSE • FBS • Ventouse and midcavity forceps
Postpartum	Maintain factor VIII/IX levels of >0.5 iu/mL for at least 3 days following a straightforward vaginal delivery and 5 days following instrumental delivery or C/S. Continue TXA postnatally until lochia is normal. Avoid VTE prophylaxis if factor VIII/IX levels < 0.6 iu/mL.	

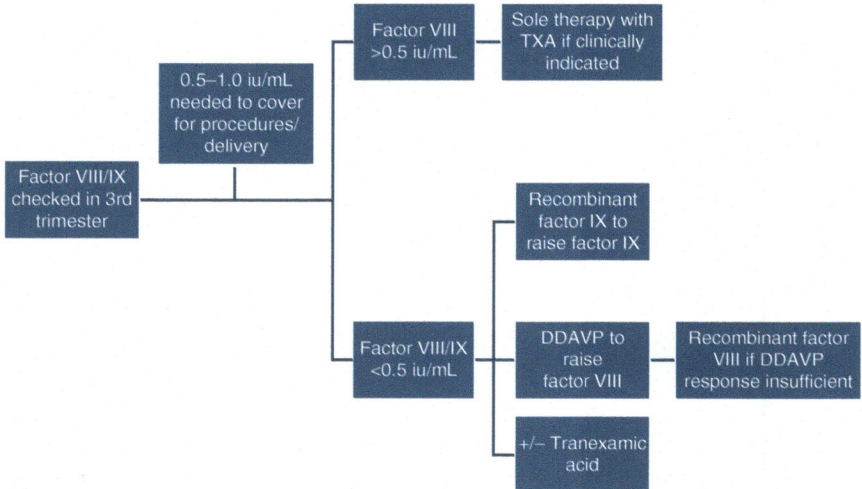

FIGURE 6.10   Algorithm for management of haemophilia in pregnancy.

Von Willibrand's Disease

See **Table 6.11** and **Figure 6.11**.

TABLE 6.11

Management of Von Willebrand's Disease in Pregnancy, Labour and Postnatally

Antenatal	The mode of delivery should be guided by obstetric indications. Aim for spontaneous labour and normal vaginal delivery to minimise risk of intervention.
Peripartum	Clotting factors should be given as close to delivery as possible Check plasma clotting factors before and after infusion and following delivery. DDAVP has antidiuretic effects; therefore, fluid restrict to 1L /24 hours to avoid hyponatraemia. Avoid DDAVP if PET. Patients with type 2B VWD may develop thrombocytopenia following DDAVP treatment.
Intrapartum	Regional anaesthesia depends on type of VWD: *Type 1*: Can be offered if factor levels are normal *Type 2*: Can be offered if factor levels are 0.5 iu/mL (this may be difficult to achieve in Type 2) *Type 3*: Avoid Avoid IM injections and NSAIDs if VWD/factor VIII levels <0.5 iu/mL	For fetuses at risk of having type 2 or 3 VWD, avoid • FSE • FBS • ECV • Ventouse • Midcavity forceps
Postpartum	Maintain VWF/factor VIII levels of >0.5 iu/mL for at least 3 days following a straightforward vaginal delivery and 5 days following instrumental delivery or C/S Continue TXA postnatally until lochia is normal

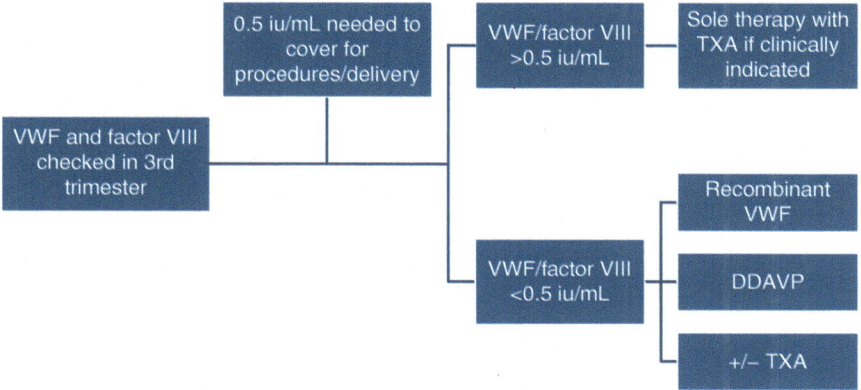

FIGURE 6.11   Algorithm for management of von Willebrand's disease in pregnancy.

Delivery Following intrauterine demise (IUD)

Diagnosis

- Auscultation or CTG are not adequate for diagnosis.
- A real-time scan is needed.
- Confirmation by a 2nd practitioner wherever possible.
- Low sensitivity of US to identify a placental abruption.

Timing of Delivery

- >85% of women with an IUD will labour spontaneously within three weeks of diagnosis
- If labour is delayed beyond 48hours, twice weekly testing for disseminated intravascular coagulation (DIC) is advised

A short delay is acceptable if

1. She is physically well

                    +

2. Membranes are intact

                    +

3. There is no laboratory evidence of DIC

Expedite delivery if there is evidence of

1. Sepsis
2. PET
3. Placental abruption
4. ROM

COUNSELLING

A physically well woman with intact membranes and no evidence of DIC is unlikely to come to physical harm if they delay labour for a short period, but

- There is a 10% risk of DIC at four weeks and this increases from the time of fetal death onwards.
- Evidence suggests greater anxiety in women who delay labour for longer intervals.
- The value of postmortem may reduce with time.
- The appearance of the baby may deteriorate with time.

Mode of Delivery

- Vaginal delivery is recommended for most women.
- Mifepristone and prostaglandin (PG) are usually first line for IOL.

Induction of Labour

- RCOG advises IOL with mifepristone + prostaglandin (PG) (e.g. misoprostol).
- There is no agreed standard regime so follow local guidance.

VBAC IOL

- Consultant obstetrician should council patient on VBAC IOL risks.
- RCOG recommends up to 600 mg mifepristone in an attempt to reduce misoprostol use/dose.

COUNSELLING

1x LSCS: PG considered acceptably safe but not without risk.
2x LSCS: The absolute risk of PG is only a little higher than for 1x LSCS.
>2x LSCS or atypical scars: The safety of IOL is unknown

Assessment

Review of AN Notes

Hx of PET, placental abruption, infection or prior SB?

Review of growth scans

SGA? (Think PET)

History

- Symptoms of PET?
- History of leaking PV?
- Abdo pain?
- Risk factors for placental abruption?

Examination

- *PA*: Woody uterus? (Think placental abruption.)
- *PS*: Sterile speculum examination if SROM?

Observations

- Febrile and tachycardic? (Think sepsis.)
- Hypertensive? (Think PET.)
- Shocked? (Think placental abruption.)

Investigations (as appropriate)

- Bloods
- Urine dip
- Blood cultures

Algorithm for the Diagnosis and Initial Management

See **Figure 6.12**.

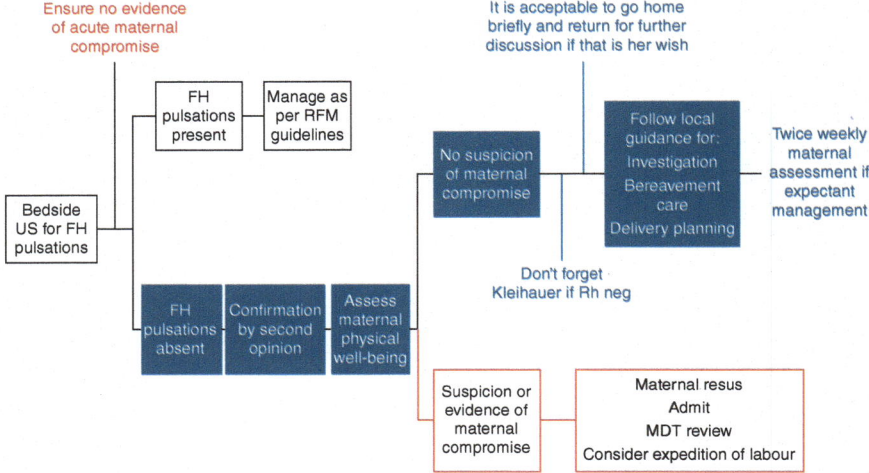

FIGURE 6.12   Algorithm for the diagnosis and initial management of patient with an intrauterine demise.

ANTIBIOTICS

Routine antibiotic prophylaxis should not be used.

Intrapartum antibiotic prophylaxis for women colonised with group B streptococcus is not indicated.

Women with sepsis should be treated with intravenous broad-spectrum antibiotic therapy (including antichlamydial agents).

ANALGESIA

Diamorphine should be used in preference to pethidine.

Regional anaesthesia should be available for women with an IUD.

Assessment for DIC and sepsis should be undertaken before administering regional anaesthesia. Women should be offered an opportunity to meet with an obstetric anaesthetist.

OBSERVATIONS

Once labour has commenced, perform observations as per normal labour.

Women undergoing VBAC should be closely monitored for features of scar rupture.

AUGMENTATION

Oxytocin augmentation can be used for VBAC, but the decision should be made by a consultant obstetrician.

SECOND STAGE

Babies who have died often deliver slowly due to absent tone.
Small premature breech babies can have a slow head delivery.

THIRD STAGE

If a baby has remained in utero for several weeks following IUD or a placental abruption is suspected, the mother has an increased PPH risk.
Other contributing factors are blood test confirming infection or clotting difficulties.
Cannulation and active management is advised.
Anecdotally retained placenta is more common with very early gestational births.

POSTPARTUM

Women should be routinely assessed for thromboprophylaxis; IUD carries a VTE score of 1.
Thromboprophylaxis with LMWH should be discussed with a haematologist if the woman has DIC.
Dopamine agonists should not be given to women with hypertension or pre-eclampsia.
Oestrogens should not be used to suppress lactation.

Hypertension in Labour

General Principles

- IOL should be considered >37/40 for hypertensive disorders in pregnancy.
- If IOL is performed for maternal PET in a preterm baby, manage the baby as per PTL.
- Severe PET carries a risk of maternal death via intracerebral haemorrhage and acute respiratory distress syndrome (ARDS). As such, intrapartum blood pressure control and fluid balance management are critical:
  - Hourly BP monitoring < BP < 160/110
  - 15-minute BP monitoring if BP >160/110
  - Input/output charting
  - Fluid restriction (80 mL/hour in severe PET)
  - Catheterisation

- Continue anti-hypertensives during labour.
- Test bloods for platelets, U+Es, LFTs and a coagulation screen if worsening of BP or development of proteinuria or symptoms of PET.
- Administer MgSO4 for eclampsia prevention if BP uncontrollable, worsening symptoms or worsening blood results.
- Empirical omeprazole as patient is at increased risk of requiring C/S
- Perform cCTG.
- Antihypertensives and magnesium sulphate may affect fetal heart rate, reducing variability and reactivity.
- *Analgesia*: Epidural may be recommended because it causes vasodilation which reduces blood pressure.
  - *NB*: If PET, avoid fluid preload prior to epidural due to fluid balance considerations.
  - Ensure platelet count allows for epidural.

Second Stage

- The duration of the 2nd stage should not be routinely limited beyond general timeframes, providing BP remains controlled.
- However, there is a low threshold for expedition of delivery, particularly if BP worsens with pushing.

Third Stage

- Active management of the third stage is advised (40 units syntocinon should be given as a concentrated infusion to reduce fluid overload – e.g. 40 units in 50mLs 0.9% normal saline at a rate of 12.5mLs/hour)
- Ergometrine should not be given as this will elevate blood pressure further.
- General anaesthetic should be avoided where possible as intubation may cause hypertension and laryngeal oedema.

Diabetes in Labour

General Principles

- Diabetes is not an indication for routine C/S.
- Diabetes is not independently a contra-indication to VBAC but incidence of large for gestational age (LFGA) is increased.
- Diabetic women are advised to give birth in obstetric units.
- Basic labour care is the same as any other labour but with additional monitoring of maternal blood glucose levels.

- 3rd trimester US assessment of fetal size is not always accurate. Even in the absence of an elevated EFW, be alert to the possibility of macrosomia if there is evidence of slow progress. Prepare for a shoulder dystocia if intervention by operative vaginal delivery is indicated for delay in the 2nd stage.

NICE (2015) advises the following intrapartum monitoring of blood glucose:

- Monitor capillary blood glucose hourly, target 4–7 mmol/L.
- An IV dextrose and insulin infusion should be considered from labour onset for women with type 1 diabetes or those whose blood glucose falls outside the normal range.
- Stable diabetic women may be fine with fluid and a light diet.
- If general anaesthetic is required, monitor blood glucose every 30 minutes until conscious.

7

Caesarean Birth

Indications for Caesarean Section

Recommend Caesarean Section (C/S) for

- ☑ Term singleton breech or transverse lie (if external cephalic version (ECV) failed/declined/contraindicated)
- ☑ Twin pregnancy where first twin is breech
- ☑ Maternal HIV with viral load >400 copies/mL (regardless of retroviral therapy)
- ☑ Concurrent HIV and Hep C
- ☑ Primary genital herpes in 3rd trimester
- ☑ Complete placenta praevia, or low-lying placenta (leading edge <2 cm from internal os)
- ☑ Maternal diabetes with estimated fetal weight (EFW) >4.5 kg
- ☑ Previous major shoulder dystocia

Maternal Request for C/S

- ① Women requesting C/S with no clinical indication should be seen in a designated birth choices clinic.
- ① Her ideas, concerns and expectations surrounding birth should be explored in detail.
- ① She should be carefully and non-judgementally counselled regarding all risks and benefits of C/S and vaginal birth.
- ① Facilitate reasonable arrangements that may make a trial of vaginal delivery acceptable.

DO NOT Routinely Offer Planned C/S for

- ☒ Twin pregnancy with first twin cephalic
- ☒ Preterm birth
- ☒ Small for gestational age (SGA) baby

DOI: 10.1201/9781003508151-7

☒ HIV positive woman on highly active antiretroviral therapy (HAART) therapy with viral load <400 copies/mL

☒ HIV woman on any retroviral therapy with viral load <50 copies/mL

☒ Maternal Hepatitis B or Hepatitis C infection

☒ Recurrent genital herpes at term

☒ BMI >50

☒ Diabetes in pregnancy without evidence of macrosomia

Preparing for C/S

Counselling

- The proposed benefit, potential risks and alternative procedures or methods should be explained.

Consent

- Written consent should be taken in advance of an elective procedure, following a shared discussion.
- This can also be done in an emergency setting when an emergency procedure becomes indicated.
- There are some situations (e.g. category 1 C/S) in which verbal consent is sufficient.
- Royal College of Obstetricians and Gynaecologists (RCOG) consent advice (2022) compares the risk of planned C/S with the risk of vaginal birth.

Timing

- For an elective caesarean section (EL C/S) identify the optimum gestation at which delivery is required; communicate any pre-operative instructions (fasting, discontinuation of heparin, etc.); and consider the need for optimisation (e.g. steroid administration, anaesthetic review, etc.).
- For an emergency caesarean section (Em C/S) communicate the urgency of the procedure using the established classification system (**Table 7.1**).

TABLE 7.1

Classification of Urgency of Procedure

Category	Description
1	Immediate threat to the life of the woman or fetus
2	Maternal or fetal compromise that is not immediately life threatening
3	No maternal or fetal compromise but needs early delivery
4	Delivery timed to suit woman or staff

Procedure

GENERAL SURGICAL PRINCIPLES

- Maintain a sterile operating field.
- Maintain adequate exposure.
- Keep tissue handling to a minimum.
- Avoid unnecessary dissection and trauma.
- Achieve haemostasis.
- Anticipate problems/complications.

SKIN INCISION

- A low transverse skin incision is preferred; there is less pain and lower risk of dehiscence, and it is cosmetically more appealing.
  1. Pfannenstiel – transverse curved abdominal incision 3 cm above pubic symphysis
  2. Joel–Cohen – straight incision 3 cm below the line that joins the anterior superior iliac spines (ASIS)
- Enter through a previous scar where possible.
- A vertical midline incision will need to be considered if access to the upper uterus is required.

ENTRY TO ABDOMEN

- Modified Joel–Cohen entry – blunt dissection of tissue layers with fingers – reduces operating time and reduces post-op febrile morbidity
- Sharp dissection if blunt is not possible

BLADDER REFLECTION

- Open visceral peritoneum over the lower uterine segment and separate from lower uterine segment (LUS).
- Displace bladder inferiorly with Doyen's retractor.
- Take care in women with previous lower section caesarean section (LSCS), as bladder likely to be adherent to LUS.

UTERINE INCISION

- Correct any rotation of uterus and make transverse incision 1–2 cm below upper margin of LUS.
- In women with previous LSCS, uterine incision should be as high as possible in LUS to avoid need to dissect bladder.
- If extending the incision bluntly, avoid downward tearing as there is a risk of trauma to vagina, bladder base and broad ligament.
- If further extension is required, a J incision is preferable to an inverted T.

- In some instances, a classical incision is preferred; transverse lie with prelabour rupture of membranes (PROM; especially if fetal back is inferior), large cervical fibroid, preterm delivery with poorly formed LUS, placenta praevia with large vessels in LUS, severe adhesions limiting access to LUS, planned caesarean hysterectomy, invasive placenta, perimortem C/S.

DELIVERY OF THE BABY

- Insert hand between fetal head and LUS. Remove Doyen's retractor and deliver in OT position through uterine incision with gentle lateral flexion and fundal pressure from the surgical assistant.
- See troubleshooting (below) for more guidance on delivery of a deeply impacted fetal head at C/S.
- In non-cephalic presentation, deliver the buttocks in the same way as described for the head. The same manoeuvres are then employed as per vaginal breech delivery.
- In non-longitudinal lies (especially preterm), identify and deliver a foot if the head/buttocks are not easily accessible. Gentle traction to the foot will then result in the buttocks becoming accessible and delivery can proceed as per breech.
- Delayed cord clamping should be employed unless immediate fetal resuscitation is required.

DELIVERY OF THE PLACENTA

- Oxytocin bolus should be given at time of birth of anterior shoulder to aid placental delivery.
- Await placental separation and delivery by controlled cord traction (CCT). (Manual removal is associated with increased blood loss, endometritis and rhesus isosensitisation.)
- Check uterine cavity to ensure that it is empty and monitor uterine tone.

UTERINE CLOSURE

- Close LUS in two layers with continuous polyfilament sutures (e.g. Vicryl/polysorb)
- First layer – Suture the inner two thirds of the myometrium, excluding the decidua.
- Second layer – invert the wound edges and suture to cover first layer.
- Check for haemostasis at the uterine incision without holding it under any tension. Haemostatic sutures (e.g. figure of 8 sutures) may be required for bleeding points.
- A classical uterine incision should be closed in three layers (interrupted sutures for first two layers and a monofilament for the third layer to prevent adhesions).

ABDOMINAL CLOSURE

- Ensure adequate haemostasis before abdominal closure and consider use of a drain if indicated (bleeding disorder, anticoagulated, difficult surgery). If a drain is used it should be soft, large-bore and non-suction (e.g. Robinsons).
- Check adnexal organs and bladder for any signs of injury.
- Check rectus sheath for any buttonholes.
- Visceral and parietal peritoneum do not need to be closed.
- Rectus sheath should be closed with number 1 polyfilament suture. If maternal body mass index (BMI) is raised, then looped polydiaxone suture (PDS) should be considered for sheath closure.
- If subcutaneous fat is >2 cm thick, then this layer should be closed.
- Skin closure should be with an absorbable monofilament suture using continuous subcuticular sutures. In women with raised BMI or risk of poor wound healing, then non-absorbable sutures or skin staples can be considered.
- PICO dressing or equivalent should be considered in patients with raised BMI, diabetes or other risk factors for poor wound healing.

POST-OP CONSIDERATIONS

- Document surgical procedure, measured blood loss and post-op plan
- Take umbilical cord gas measurements
- Assess thrombosis risk (emergency LSCS is an intermediate risk factor for venous thromboembolism [VTE]). Local scoring systems should be used, and low-molecular-weight heparin (LMWH) prescribed accordingly.
- Plan for removal of indwelling catheter.
- Plan for removal of any drains.
- Inform patient if there are any contraindications to consideration of a vaginal birth after caesarean (VBAC) in subsequent pregnancies, and ensure this is documented in the notes.

Troubleshooting: Deeply Impacted Fetal Head

C/S in late labour or at full dilatation with reduced liquor and an engaged fetal head is a difficult procedure and carries a higher risk of complications for both mother and baby.

The *National Sentinel Caesarean Section Audit Report* (Thomas et al. 2000) recommends a consultant presence when C/S is performed at full dilatation.

A careful abdominal palpation and vaginal examination should be performed to assess position and engagement of the fetal head and any excessive moulding of the fetal head to help predict difficulty in delivery of the baby at C/S. See also **Table 7.2**.

TABLE 7.2

Risk Factors for Difficult Delivery at LSCS

- Unsuccessful instrumental delivery
- Deep transverse arrest
- Arrest in occipital-posterior (OP) position
- Cephalopelvic disproportion

Complications

See **Table 7.3**.

TABLE 7.3

Potential Complications of Caesarean Section with a Deeply Impacted Fetal Head

Mother	Baby
• High rate of extension of the uterine incision	• Difficulty delivering head
• Obstetric haemorrhage	• Delay between knife to skin and delivery
• Urinary tract injury	• Skull fractures
• Damage to uterine vessels	• Cephalhaematoma
• Increased length of hospital stays	• Subgaleal haematoma

- Uterine extensions can occur due to excessive manipulation that may be required to deliver the fetal head when the lower uterine segment is already thin, oedematous and overstretched.
- Difficulty in delivering the fetal head, leading to delay between uterine incision and delivery in an already compromised fetus.
- Direct fetal trauma resulting from attempts at extracting a deeply engaged head from the pelvis.

Techniques for Delivery of a Deeply Engaged Head

Difficulty in delivering the fetal head may arise due to a number of reasons:

1. Lack of space between bony pelvis and fetal head
2. Fetal head deeply engaged in pelvis, making it difficult to reach the occiput to achieve adequate flexion for delivery
3. Fetal malposition, making it difficult to reach the occiput
4. Raised maternal BMI or other factors making access to the pelvis challenging

Techniques for Delivery of a Deeply Impacted Fetal Head

INITIAL TECHNIQUES

- Ensure you have the table at the lowest height possible and stand on a step if required so you can be high above the patient.
- Ask the anaesthetist for head-down tilt of the table.
- Give a utero-relaxant (terbutaline/GTN).
- Use your non-dominant hand on the fetal head to allow greater upwards force to dislodge fetal head from pelvis.

ELEVATING FETAL HEAD VAGINALLY BY ASSISTANT

- Pressure on fetal head should be with the palmar aspect of 3 or 4 fingers.
- This should be performed only by a trained assistant.
- It may lead to significant delay in uterine incision to delivery time.
- Can be associated with fetal skull trauma due to uncontrolled or focal force.

FETAL PILLOW (SEE SEPARATE BOX AND FIGURE 7.1)

- This is designed to elevate fetal head out of the pelvis in a non-traumatic manner, as an alternative to assistant dislodging the head vaginally.
- Initial studies were promising but some have now been questioned as to their reliability and so further evidence is required prior to their use being recommended as routine.
- Method for insertion is outlined below.

REVERSE BREECH EXTRACTION

- Deliver baby's feet or buttocks through the uterine incision first.
- Once body is delivered, baby's head can be lifted out of pelvis.
- Uterine extensions are common, and so incision can be extended into a J-shaped or inverted T prior to reverse breech extraction.

Method for Inserting Fetal Pillow to Aid in Elevation of the Fetal Head

Fetal Pillow (see Figure 7.1)
Place patient in lithotomy position.
↓
Apply obstetric cream or lubricant to the balloon.
↓
Hold the deflated balloon device like folded wings between the thumb and the finger, making sure that the tube attachment is at the inferior end.
↓
Insert this in the vagina and place it behind the fetal head.
↓

(Continued)

Let the device unfold to lay flat, with the deflated surface in direct contact with the fetal head and push it posteriorly towards the sacral bone of mum.
↓
Place patient's legs flat on the operating table.*
↓
Inflate the balloon with normal saline or water using a large 60 mL syringe, to a total of 180 mL.**
↓
Close the tap to ensure balloon remains inflated.
↓
Proceed with LSCS.
↓
Deflate balloon following delivery of the baby.
↓
Remove device at the end of the procedure by hooking a finger over the plate and gently removing from the vagina.

* This is essential prior to inflating the balloon to ensure that it does not become dislodged during inflation.

** Never inflate with air, maximum saline volume 300 mL.

Fetal pillow is contraindicated in the presence of active genital infection

STEP 1 INSERTION

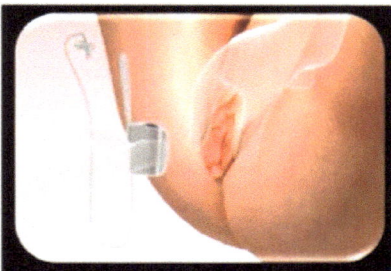

- Bi-fold the device in two
- Lubricate device
- Insert vaginally ensuring the balloon surface is in contact with the fetal head

STEP 2 PLACEMENT

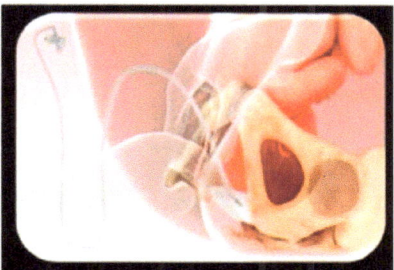

- Push the device as posteriorly as possible, towards sacrum
- Placement is similar to a posterior ventouse cup

STEP 3 LEGS FLAT

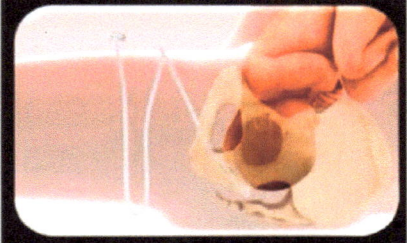

- Lay the legs flat on the operating table - otherwise it can be expelled or displaced if legs are open

STEP 4 INFLATE

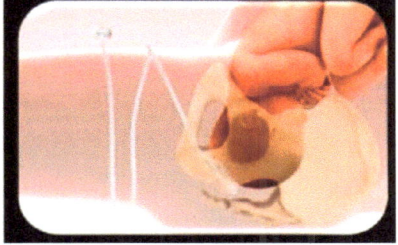

- Inflate with 180 mL of saline using the 60 mL syringe provided - Three full syringes

FIGURE 7.1   Fetal pillow procedure. (With permission from CooperSurgical.com.)

Complication: Excessive Intra-Operative Bleeding

*Consideration of risk factors (**Table 7.4**) prior to the procedure allows pre-emptive measures to be taken, such as valid group and screen sample, suitable cross-matched blood, cell salvage set up and a senior obstetrician present. If there is a significant risk of post-partum haemorrhage (PPH) then prophylactic uterotonics should be given intra-operatively.*

> **TABLE 7.4**
>
> Risk Factors for Excessive Bleeding at LSCS
>
> - Raised maternal BMI
> - Maternal bleeding disorders or anticoagulation
> - Large for gestational age (LFGA) or polyhydramnios
> - Prolonged or augmented labour
> - LSCS at full dilatation
> - Multiple pregnancy

Techniques in the Case of Excessive Intraoperative Bleeding

INITIAL TECHNIQUES

- If bleeding is due to uterine atony, then uterine massage, bimanual compression and uterotonics should be given as per management of PPH following vaginal birth.
- If bleeding is surgical/traumatic, then clamp any large bleeding vessels early (can even be done prior to delivery of baby and/or placenta) to minimise surgical blood loss.

EXTERIORISATION OF UTERUS

- Exteriorising the uterus often allows a better view and better access to bleeding points.
- It also allows visualisation of the posterior aspect of uterus in case of any bleeding from an extended incision
- Ensure to inform patient and anaesthetist prior to exteriorising the uterus.
- Can lead to hypothermia, so cover uterus with a large swab soaked in warm saline.

LIGATION OF UTERINE ARTERIES (FIGURE 7.2)

- In uterine bleeding, ligation of the uterine arteries will result in immediate and substantial slowing of blood loss (as they are responsible for 90% of uterine blood supply).
- After exteriorising the uterus, use a 1 or 0 polyfilament suture; pass a suture through the myometrium just below and lateral to the angle of uterine incision, through the posterior wall of the uterus, and back through the avascular triangle of the broad ligament. Tie securely and repeat on the other side.

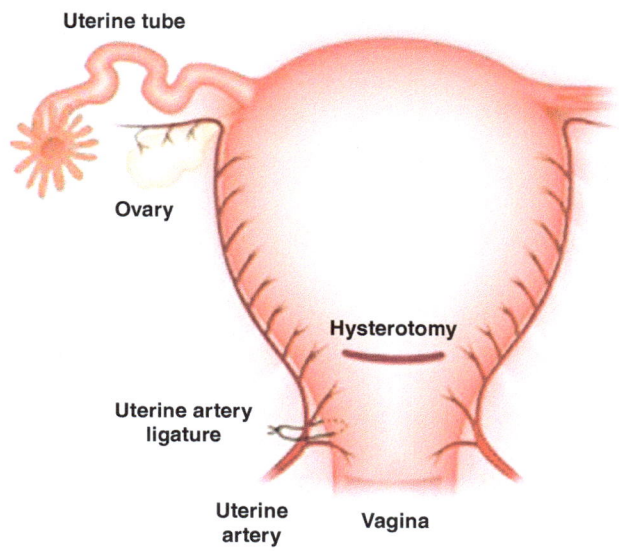

FIGURE 7.2 Ligation of uterine arteries. (With permission from Osanan GC et al., Non-conservative and Conservative Surgical Management of PPH, *Glob Libr Women's Med* 2021.)

INTRA-UTERINE BALLOON TAMPONADE

- Bakri balloon and Rouche balloon are the most commonly used intra-uterine balloons.
- Pass tubing of balloon into uterine incision and down through cervix for an assistant to gently pull through the vagina.
- Place balloon correctly in uterine cavity, with tip of tube close to fundus.
- Close the uterine incision prior to inflating the balloon, to avoid piercing the inflated balloon with a needle.
- Inflate balloon with required amount of saline to form a tamponade.
- A vaginal pack often needs to be inserted to ensure the balloon is not expelled vaginally at the time of inflating
- Ensure you document plan for timing of deflation and removal of balloon (usually 12 hours post-op if no signs of bleeding).

B-LYNCH SUTURE (FIGURE 7.3)

Use a size 0 polyfilament suture on a large round bodied needle:

- Insert suture just below angle of uterine incision in the lower segment on one side, and then back out through anterior uterine wall just above the incision.

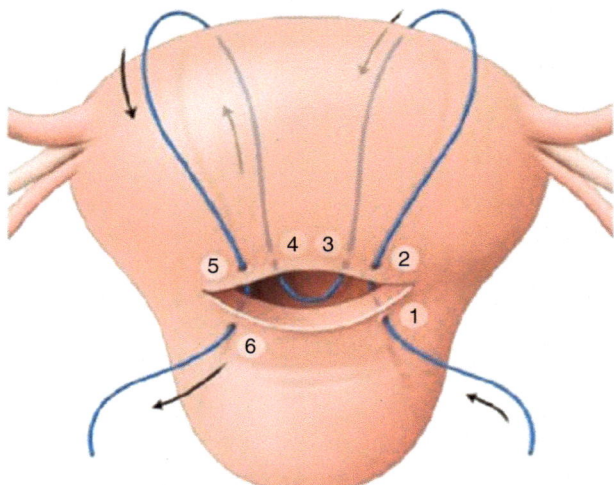

FIGURE 7.3   B-Lynch brace suture. (With permission from Bouchghoul H et al., Uterine-sparing surgical procedures to control postpartum hemorrhage, *Am J Obstet Gynecol* 2024;230/3:S1066–S1075.e4.)

- Loop the suture over the fundus and into the posterior uterine wall at the same level as the incision.
- Pass the suture horizontally inside the uterine cavity, and then back out through the posterior wall level with the angle of the incision on the other side.
- Loop the suture over the fundus again so it passes over the anterior aspect of the uterus.
- Pass the needle through the anterior uterine wall just above the level of the incision, and then back out through the anterior lower segment below the incision.
- Pull the suture tight whilst the surgical assistant is manually compressing the uterus (to avoid the suture cutting through the myometrium) and tie to secure.

Some obstetricians will opt to pass the needle through the fundus to secure the 'loops' at the fundus.

SURGICEL

- It can be applied to 'raw' or 'oozing' areas which are not amenable to suturing.
- It is particularly common where excessive dissection was required due to adhesions.
- It is particularly common on lower uterine segment.

- It has clotting factors embedded in it to promote coagulation where applied.
- Simply lay over the oozing areas prior to closing.
- Ensure that its use is documented in the surgical notes, as it can mimic a haematoma/collection on CT scan if patient goes on to have this post-operatively.

 ## Complication: Suspected Visceral Injury (Table 7.5)

General Principles

- Ensure adequate access, exposure and lighting.
- Use an additional assistant if access is challenging.
- Consider use of retractors to improve access.
- If access is poor, extend abdominal incision early.

TABLE 7.5

Risk factors for visceral injury during LSCS

- Category 1 LSCS or rapid entry of abdominal cavity
- Previous LSCS or other previous abdominal surgery leading to intra-abdominal adhesions
- Previous pelvic inflammatory disease or infection causing adhesions
- Poor access or vision of operative site

Management of Visceral Injures at Caesarean Section

BLADDER INJURY

- Risk is 1:1000; it more common in VBAC. Usually occurs upon entry if first LSCS but may be at time of bladder reflection at repeat LSCS.
- High suspicion if difficult entry/multiple adhesions. Test with methylene blue if suspected, as prognosis better if recognised intraoperatively and repaired.
- Should be repaired by a senior or a urologist if complex or suspicion of ureteric involvement.
- Post-op, require indwelling catheter for 10–14 days. Perform a cystogram to confirm bladder integrity, and then remove catheter.

URETERIC INJURY

- Missed intra-operatively in 70% of cases.
- Most common type of injury is transection (can occur when there is extension of uterine incision into the broad ligament) or ligation by a suture.
- There is risk of inclusion within a suture during attempts at haemostasis because of close proximity to uterine arteries.

- There is a high index of suspicion required if injury suspected.
- Management depends on injury and location – may require stenting, re-implantation of ureter into bladder, re-anastamosis of transected ureter. Needs urologist for repair.

BOWEL INJURY

Bowel may be adherent to anterior abdominal wall (particularly if previous mid-line incision) and may be damaged during peritoneal entry or division of adhesions. May also be damaged during uterine closure as loops of bowel can be included within the sutures posterior to the uterus.

Thermal bowel injury is difficult to spot and may lead to perforation secondary to necrosis after 48–72 hours.

Primary repair should be attempted for almost all injuries, by a surgeon.

If not recognised intra-operatively, bowel perforation will usually present with intra-abdominal sepsis.

8

Operative Vaginal Delivery

Rationale

Operative intervention is used to shorten the second stage of labour. It may be indicated for conditions of the fetus or of the mother (**Tables 8.1** and **8.2**).

TABLE 8.1

Indications for Operative Vaginal Delivery

Fetal	Expedite birth	Presumed fetal compromise
Obstetric	Expedite birth	Inadequate progress Maternal exhaustion
Maternal	Shorten second stage	Maternal medical conditions where Valsalva manoeuvre should be avoided: • Heart disease class III or IV • Hypertensive crises • Myasthenia Gravis • Spinal cord injury • Proliferative retinopathy

TABLE 8.2

When to Expedite Birth for Lack of Progress

	With Regional Anaesthesia After	Without Regional Anaesthesia After
Nullip	3 hours (Total of active + Passive 2nd stage)	2 hours
Multip	2 hours (Total of active + Passive 2nd stage)	1 hour

* A retrospective cohort study of 15,759 nulliparous women demonstrated that maternal morbidity increased significantly after 3 hours of the second stage and further increased after 4 hours.

DOI: 10.1201/9781003508151-8

Classification

See **Table 8.3**.

TABLE 8.3

Classification of Operative Vaginal Delivery

	PA	PV	Subclassification Based on Rotation
High*	>2/5	Above spines	
Mid	1/5	Spines to <+2	Rotation of ≤45° from occipito-anterior (OA)
			Rotation of >45° including occipital-posterior (OP)
Low	0/5	+2 to pelvic floor	Rotation of ≤45° from OA
			Rotation of >45° including OP
Outlet**	0/5	On perineum	Sagittal suture is in the A-P diameter (either OA or OP)

* Not included in classification as not recommended to perform OVD if head is >2/5 palpable abdominally, or above the spines vaginally

** Fetal scalp visible without parting the labia

Instrument Choice

The operator should choose the instrument most appropriate to the clinical circumstances and their level of skill.

Location

Operative vaginal births that have a higher risk of failure should be considered a trial and conducted in a place where immediate recourse to caesarean section (C/S) can be undertaken.

Higher rates of failure are associated with the following factors, and a trial of instrumental delivery in theatre is recommended:

1. Body mass index (BMI) >30
2. Estimated fetal weight (EFW) >4000 g (or clinically big baby)
3. OP (or other position requiring rotation)
4. Mid-cavity
5. Factors which inhibit a rapid transfer to theatre

Cautions and Contraindications

See **Tables 8.4** and **8.5**.

TABLE 8.4

Contra-Indications and Cautions of OVD

	Absolute	Relative	Caution
Vacuum extraction	<32+0 Face presentation Breech presentation Assisted birth under general anaesthesia		32+0–36+0
All OVD	Prior to full dilatation	Fetal bleeding disorder Fetal fracture risk (e.g. osteogenesis imperfecta)	Blood-borne viral infections of the mother

TABLE 8.5

Contra-Indication/Caution

Vacuum extraction <32+0	There is risk of cephalohaematoma, intracranial haemorrhage, subgaleal haemorrhage and neonatal jaundice.
Vacuum extraction 32+0–36+0	There is insufficient safety data. Use with caution due to risk of subgaleal and intracranial haemorrhage.
Fetal bleeding disorder Fetal fracture risk	Be aware that delivery of deeply impacted head at caesarean also carries risks
Blood-borne viral infections of the mother	It is sensible to avoid difficult operative delivery where there is an increased chance of fetal abrasion or scalp trauma

Complications

See **Table 8.6**.

TABLE 8.6

Rates of Complications for Vacuum Extraction vs Forceps

	Vacuum Extraction	Forceps
Failure	Higher	
Cephalohaematoma	Higher	
Retinal haemorrhage	Higher	
Maternal worries about baby	Higher	
Significant maternal perineal and vaginal trauma		Higher
Delivery by C/S	Equal	
Low 5-minute Apgar scores	Equal	
Need for phototherapy	Equal	

Source: Johanson, 2000.

Note: The relative merits of vacuum extraction and forceps have been evaluated in a Cochrane systematic review of ten randomised controlled trials, involving primiparous and multiparous women.

Sequential Instruments

- The use of sequential instruments is associated with an **increased risk of trauma to the baby**:
  - The risk of intracranial haemorrhage is 1:256 for sequential instruments vs 1:334 for failed forceps proceding C/S.
  - Neonatal intracranial and subgaleal haemorrhage are life threatening complications and the risk is significantly greater in babies exposed to attempts at delivery with sequential instruments.
  - Risk of neonatal trauma and admission to neonatal intensive care unit (NICU) is increased following more than three pulls of an instrument, and the use of sequential instruments. This risk is increased further if delivery if by C/S after a protracted attempt at vaginal delivery.
- This must be balanced against the risks of a C/S following failed vacuum extraction with the risks of forceps delivery following failed vacuum extraction.
- C/S in the second stage of labour is associated with an increased risk of major obstetric haemorrhage, prolonged hospital stays and admission of the baby to the special care baby unit compared with completed instrumental delivery.

Checklist for OVD

See **Table 8.7**.

VACUUM EXTRACTION

There are different types of ventouse cups. They are either rigid (metal) or soft (silicone) and are either anterior or posterior, depending on their design.

Application

1. Position patient in lithotomy position.
2. Lubricate cup well and insert sideways into the introitus.
3. Identify the flexion point (**Figure 8.1**).

Correct cup placement on the flexion point will ensure that head is flexed so that the smallest diameter of the fetal head is presenting.

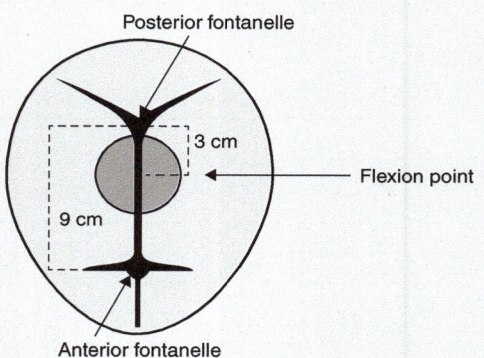

FIGURE 8.1 Flexion point. (With permission from Keriakos R et al., *Instrumental Vaginal Delivery – Back to Basics*, J Obstet Gynecol 2013;33/8:781–6.)

TABLE 8.7

Checklist for OVD

- ☐ Head is no more than 1/5th palpable abdominally.
- ☐ Cervix is fully dilated.
- ☐ Membranes are not intact.
- ☐ Presentation is vertex.
- ☐ Position of head is established.
- ☐ Caput and moulding are assessed.
- ☐ Pelvis is deemed adequate (moulding may indicate cephalo-pelvic disproportion [CPD]).
- ☐ Mother is informed and consented (for deliveries in theatre, written consent is required; for deliveries in the room, verbal consent is sufficient).
- ☐ Analgesia has been applied.
- ☐ Bladder is emptied.
- ☐ Aseptic technique

Optimal flexion is achieved when the centre of the cup is applied over the flexion point.

To avoid asynclitism, ensure cup is central over sagittal suture.

Vacuum

1. Create some vacuum (either by pumping handle if using a Kiwi, or with vacuum pump on a ventouse).
2. At a pressure of 0.2 kg/cm, check around the edges of the ventouse cup to ensure there is no entrapment of maternal vaginal tissue.
3. Increase pressure to 0.8 kg/cm.

Traction

1. Force of traction should be perpendicular and downwards, to maintain flexion in the direction of the pelvic axis.
2. Pulling hand should provide the traction, other hand should provide counter-traction with a thumb and finger on the dome of the cup to assess descent and reduce risk of cup detachment.
3. Fetal head should reach the perineum (and ventouse cup be fully visible at the introitus) with three pulls.
4. Delivery of the fetal head should occur within a further three pulls.

Removal

1. Once fetal head is delivered, release the vacuum and remove the cup prior to delivery of the body.

For essential points, note also **Table 8.8**.

TABLE 8.8

Essential Points about Ventouse Delivery

- **Abandon attempts at ventouse delivery if there is inadequate descent with traction, or if there are two detachments of the cup.**
- Ventouse cup should be applied over flexion point, centrally over the sagittal suture.
- Ensure there is no entrapment of vaginal tissue in cup before proceeding to full vacuum pressure.
- Head should reach perineum within three pulls and be delivered within a further three.
- Ventouse cup application time should not exceed 15 minutes.

ROTATIONAL VACUUM DELIVERY

See **Table 8.9**.

TABLE 8.9

Types of Cups Appropriate for Rotational Delivery

Cups that can be used for rotational delivery	Cups that cannot be used for rotational delivery
Kiwi	Silastic
Metal posterior cup	Metal anterior cup

See **Table 8.10**.

TABLE 8.10

Fetal Positions Suitable for Rotational Delivery

Fetal positions suitable for vacuum delivery	Fetal positions NOT suitable for vacuum delivery
OA	Face presentation
OP	Brow presentation
OT	Non-cephalic presentation

Method

- The cup must still be placed on the flexion point, regardless of fetal position.
- For OP position, the cup will be placed far back. Traction will then flex the head and allow some descent, and rotation will occur spontaneously as descent continues.

- The measurements on the tubing help to determine if the flexion cup is on the right place.
  - *Occipito-transverse (OT) position*: 6 cm
  - *OP position*: 11 cm
- For OT positions the cup should be placed in the MIDLINE and not laterally to one side. When the baby lies in an OT position, the flexion point is central.
- Once the cup is applied, do not try to rotate the head by twisting the cup or handle.
- Apply downward pressure as per non-rotational vacuum delivery, which encourages natural internal rotation.
- As the head flexes and descends onto the pelvic floor, it will auto-rotate into an OA position.

FORCEPS DELIVERY

Two Types of Non-Rotational Forceps

1. Low-cavity outlet forceps, e.g. Wrigleys. They are short and light and used when the head is on the perineum.
2. Mid-cavity forceps, e.g. Neville Barnes. They are used when fetal head is +2 station or higher, and when the sagittal suture is in the AP plane, or no more than 45° from the midline.

Application of Forceps

1. Apply the left blade first, when there is no uterine contraction.
2. Protect vaginal walls with right hand; hold handle of left forceps blade in left-handed pencil grip.
3. Forceps blade should be held parallel to inguinal ligament.
4. Guide forceps into position, with right thumb on pelvic curve of forceps blade.
5. Repeat the process for the right forceps blade.
6. Check that blades lock easily, and that sagittal suture is in the midline, equidistant from the blades.
7. Unlock blades until you are ready to pull, to minimise trauma to the perineum.

Traction with Forceps

1. Apply traction with contractions.
2. Pajot's manoeuvre = Downwards force, perpendicular to the handle whilst applying traction to the forceps, to maintain fetal head flexion, and delivery in the direction of the pelvic axis.

3. Delivery of the head should be achieved with three or four contractions, but **descent should be achieved with each contraction**.
4. Perform right mediolateral episiotomy at the time of crowning.
5. Once posterior fontanelle is below the symphysis pubis, elevate the forceps handles in a 'J' movement.

Removal of Forceps

Once fetal head is delivered, remove forceps blades by sliding them along fetal head. Remove the right forceps blade first, followed by the left.

For essential points about forceps delivery, see **Table 8.11**.

TABLE 8.11

Essential Points about Forceps Delivery

- Attempts at vaginal delivery should be abandoned if there is no descent with traction to correctly applied forceps.
- Forceps blades should be applied easily, without force.
- Forceps blades should lock with ease.
- Sagittal suture should lie vertically in the midline, equidistant from the blades.
- There should be space to insert a fingertip between the end of the fenestration and the fetal head.
- Attempts at vaginal delivery should be abandoned if there is no descent with traction to correctly applied forceps

---

ROTATIONAL FORCEPS DELIVERY

Rotational forceps are called Keilland's forceps. They have the following features:

1. No pelvic curve, to allow rotation without causing fetal or maternal trauma
2. Sliding lock, to allow correction of asynclitism
3. Occiput markers (bobble or small knob on the handles), to allow assessment of rotation

Application

1. The knob on the handles should always be pointed towards the fetal occiput.

Occipito-Posterior Position

Direct application: Apply blades in the same way as non-rotational forceps (see above), ensuring that the knob is pointing towards the fetal occiput.

Occipito-Transverse Position

1. *Direct application*: Anterior blade is applied first, again with the knob pointing towards the fetal occiput. Posterior blade is then passed into the sacral hollow (either directly, or at a 45° angle and then slid into the midline).
2. *Wandering application*: If there is no space anteriorly between the pubic symphysis and the fetal head, then the anterior blade can be inserted posteriorly and 'wandered' or 'swept' round into an anterior position. The posterior blade is then inserted as above.

Rotation

1. Rotation should always follow the shortest path.
2. Slide handles so that the knobs on the handles line up – this corrects any asynclitism.
3. The handles of the forceps should be held pointing downwards towards the floor, at an angle of 45° (causes upwards displacement of the fetal head so that rotation is occurring in the mid cavity, where there is more space).
4. Gentle rotation with thumb and finger should be enough force to rotate the head. If any more force than this is required, then the procedure should be abandoned.
5. Once fetal head reaches OA position, a 'clunk' is usually felt as it enters the pelvis.

Traction

1. Once fetal head is in an OA position and has entered the pelvis, traction should be performed in exactly the same manner as non-rotational forceps, described above.

PREPARING FOR OVD

- Examination
- Instrument selection
- Location selection
- Consent
- Analgesia
- Empty bladder

PERFORMING OVD

Aspectic technique

- Deflate balloon of indwelling catheter
- Assess for episiotomy – restrictive use of episiotomy recommended
- Perform operative vaginal delivery

COMPLETING OVD

- Anticipate complications – post-partum haemorrhage (PPH), shoulder dystocia.
- Assess for perineal trauma.
- Debrief patient

AFTERCARE

- Stat dose of prophylactic broad-spectrum antibiotics is recommended following all instrumental deliveries.
- Venous thromboembolism (VTE) re-assessment – mid-cavity or rotational delivery, prolonged labour and immobility are risk factors.
- Offer analgesia – non-steroidal anti-inflammatory drug (NSAID) and paracetamol
- Offer physiotherapy-directed strategies to prevent urinary incontinence.

BLADDER CARE POST OVD

- The timing and volume of the first void urine should be monitored and documented.
- A post-void residual should be measured if retention is suspected.
- Women who have had a spinal anaesthetic or an epidural that has been topped up for a trial may be at increased risk of retention and should be recommended to have an indwelling catheter in place for at least 12 hours post-delivery.
- Operative delivery, prolonged labour and epidural analgesia may predispose to postpartum urinary retention.

SUBSEQUENT DELIVERIES

- Women should be encouraged to aim for a spontaneous vaginal delivery in a subsequent pregnancy.
- The likelihood of achieving a spontaneous vaginal delivery is approximately 90%.

9

Obstetric Emergencies

Umbilical Cord Prolapse

Umbilical cord prolapse is the descent of the umbilical cord alongside or past the presenting part, in the presence of ruptured membranes; it carries a perinatal mortality rate of 91:1000. **Figure 9.1** lists risk factors for umbilical cord prolapse, and **Figure 9.2** outlines a management approach to umbilical cord prolapse.

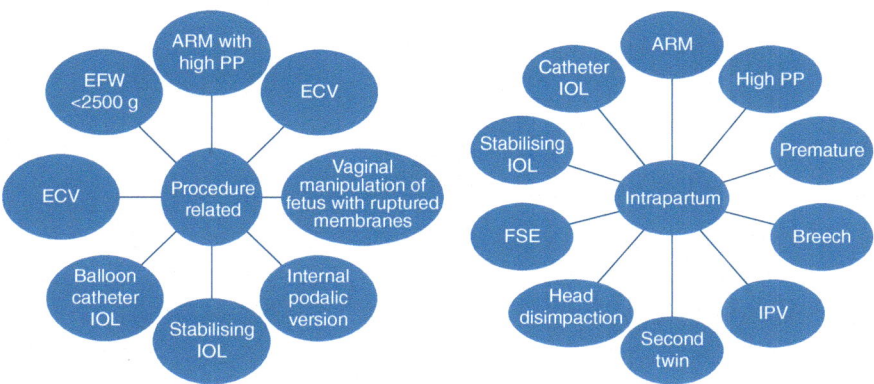

FIGURE 9.1   Risk factors.

Fetal Bradycardia

- Acute fetal bradycardia is a single prolonged deceleration lasting 3 minutes or more
- Urgent management required as fetal cord pH drops by 0.009 per minute of bradycardia to delivery.

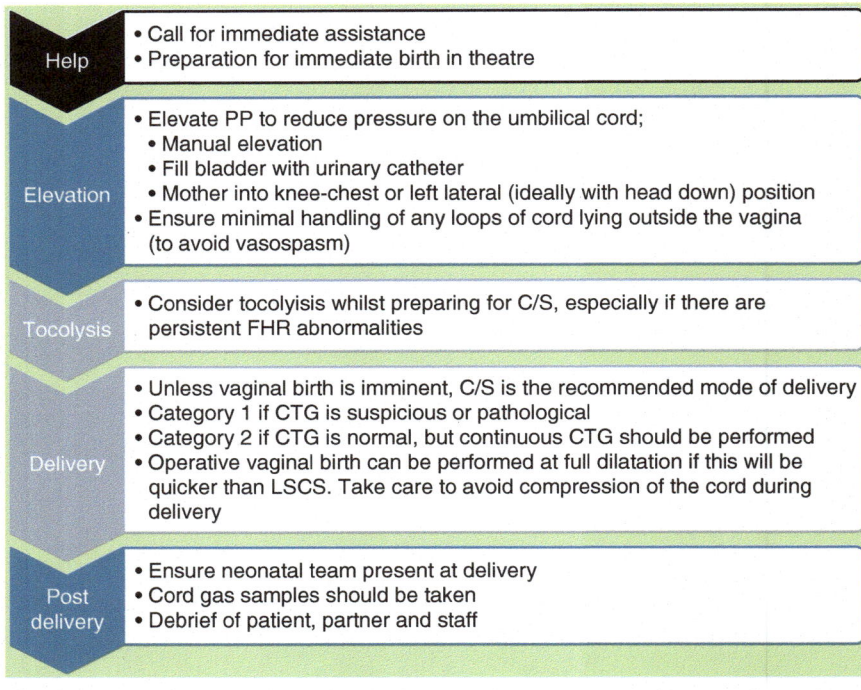

FIGURE 9.2 Management.

Causes of Acute Fetal Bradycardia

Maternal position

- Supine position can affect uterine blood flow and cord compression.
- Encourage left lateral position (or another alternative to supine).

Hypotension

- Only offer IV fluids for cardio tocograph (CTG) abnormalities if woman is hypotensive or septic.
- If secondary to epidural top-up, start IV fluids, put in left lateral and call for anaesthetic review.

Excessive contractions

- Stop or reduce oxytocin if being used.
- Offer a tocolytic (subcut terbutaline 250 µg).

Figure 9.3 Outlines a management approach to an acute fetal bradycardia.

FIGURE 9.3 Management.

Shoulder Dystocia

This is defined **as a vaginal cephalic birth that requires additional obstetric manoeuvres to release the impacted shoulder after the head has been born and routine traction employed to deliver a fetus has failed**.

It occurs when anterior fetal shoulder impacts on maternal pubic symphysis or (less commonly) posterior fetal shoulder impacts on maternal sacral promontory.

TABLE 9.1

Morbidity Associated with Shoulder Dystocia

- Brachial plexus injury
- Fracture of humerus or clavicle
- Hypoxic brain injury
- Pneumothorax
- Death

Risk Factors

Shoulder dystocia is an unpredictable event. However, there are some factors known to be associated with shoulder dystocia (**Table 9.1**; **Figure 9.4**).

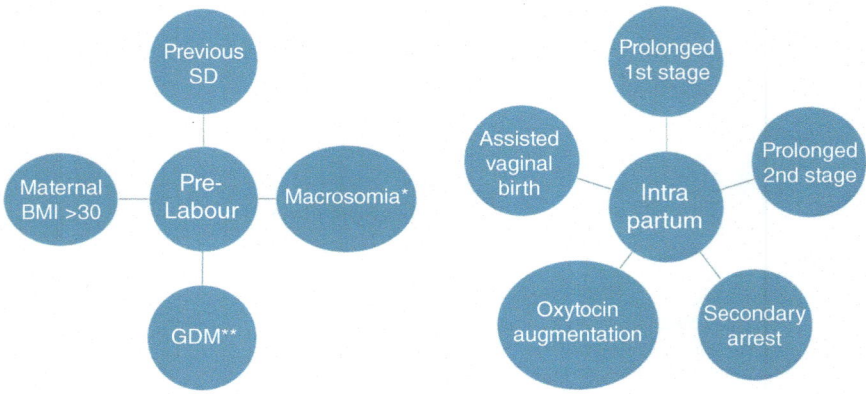

FIGURE 9.4   Risk factors for shoulder dystocia.

* Although there is a relationship between fetal size and shoulder dystocia, a large majority of babies
with a birth weight >4.5 kg does not develop shoulder dystocia, and 48% of shoulder dystocias
occur in babies who weigh less than 4 kg.
** Babies of diabetic mothers have a 2x–4x increased risk of shoulder dystocia compared to babies
of same birth weight born to non-diabetic mothers (not explained solely by macrosoamia).

Management of Shoulder Dystocia

See **Table 9.2**.

TABLE 9.2

General Measures

Management	Rationale
Perform routine traction in an axial direction.	Downward traction can cause brachial plexus injury.
Avoid fundal pressure.	Fundal pressure can cause uterine rupture.
Discourage maternal pushing.	Pushing will exacerbate impaction of the shoulders.
Bring women to end of bed or take end of bed.	It provides improved access.
Insert whole hand into posterior aspect of vagina when undertaking manoeuvres.	Most spacious part of pelvis is sacral hollow; therefore, vaginal access should be posterior.

The mnemonic 'HELPER' (**Figure 9.5**) can be used to help remember the stages of
shoulder dystocia management.

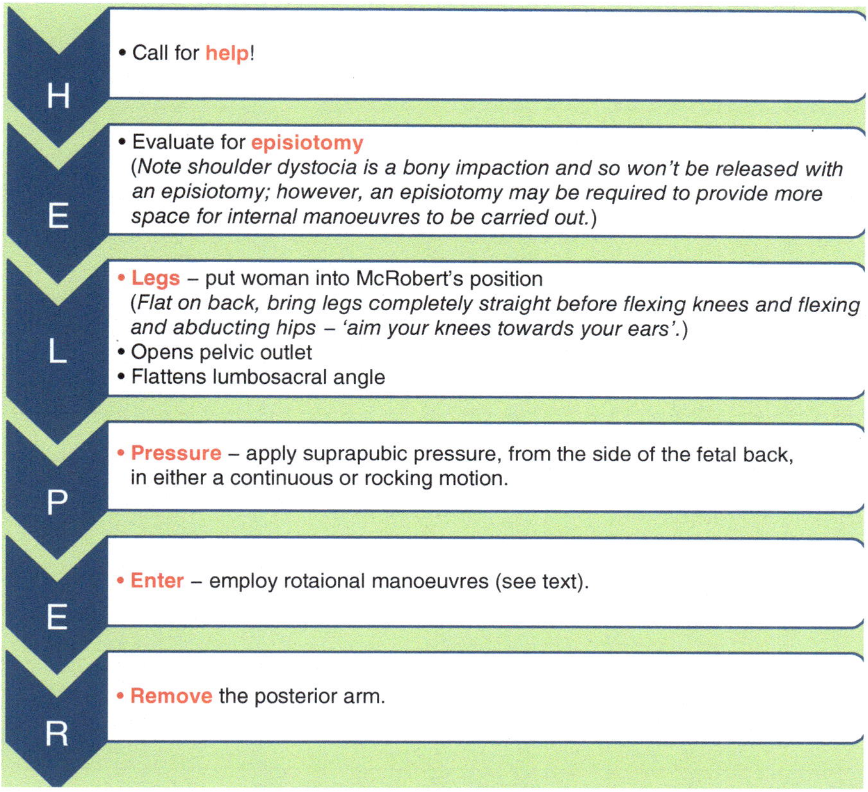

H
- Call for **help**!

E
- Evaluate for **episiotomy**
  (*Note shoulder dystocia is a bony impaction and so won't be released with an episiotomy; however, an episiotomy may be required to provide more space for internal manoeuvres to be carried out.*)

L
- **Legs** – put woman into McRobert's position
  (*Flat on back, bring legs completely straight before flexing knees and flexing and abducting hips – 'aim your knees towards your ears'.*)
- Opens pelvic outlet
- Flattens lumbosacral angle

P
- **Pressure** – apply suprapubic pressure, from the side of the fetal back, in either a continuous or rocking motion.

E
- **Enter** – employ rotaional manoeuvres (see text).

R
- **Remove** the posterior arm.

FIGURE 9.5   HELPER mnemonic.

Internal Manoeuvres

See **Tables 9.3** and **9.4**.

TABLE 9.3

Internal Manoeuvres

Manoeuvre	Description	Rationale
Suprapubic pressure	Firm constant or rocking pressure above the pubic symphysis, applied from the side of the fetal back	Dislodge impacted anterior shoulder from below the pubic symphysis
Rubin I	Push the posterior aspect of fetal anterior shoulder to fetal chest	Reduces the fetal biparietal diameter
Rubin II	Press on the posterior aspect of the anterior shoulder	Rotate shoulders into wider oblique diameter of pelvis. It will also adduct the shoulder

(Continued)

TABLE 9.3 *(Continued)*

Internal Manoeuvres

Manoeuvre	Description	Rationale
Wood's corkscrew	Press on the anterior aspect of the posterior shoulder	Rotate shoulders into wider oblique diameter of pelvis. It will also adduct the shoulders
Rubin II + Woods corkscrew	Press on posterior aspect of anterior shoulder at same time as anterior aspect of posterior shoulder	Rotate shoulders into wider oblique diameter of pelvis. It will also adduct the shoulders
Reverse Woods corkscrew	Press on posterior aspect of posterior should rotate trunk into oblique diameter of pelvis in the opposite direction to initially tried	Rotate shoulders into wider oblique diameter of pelvis. It will also adduct the shoulders

TABLE 9.4

Delivery of Posterior Arm

Manoeuvre	Description	Rationale
Deliver posterior arm.	Follow posterior arm to antecubital fossa. Apply pressure at antecubital fossa to flex. Grasp fetal wrist and withdraw posterior arm in a straight line.	Reduces the diameter of the fetal shoulder by the width of the arm, allowing you to rotate trunk into oblique diameter to bring the anterior shoulder under the pubic symphysis. (It is associated with humeral fractures.)

Note: These manoeuvres can be attempted in any order, depending on your preference. Attempt each manoeuvre for no longer than 60 seconds before moving on to the next manoeuvre. However, you can move on quicker than this if it is clear that one manoeuvre isn't going to be effective in delivering the baby.

Third Line Manoeuvres

See **Table 9.5**.

TABLE 9.5

Third Line

Manoeuvre	Description	Rationale
Cleidotomy	Fracture fetal clavicle with firm pressure in the centre.	Reduces fetal biacromial diameter
Symphysiotomy	Divide anterior fibres of symphyseal ligament.	Increases pelvic diameter
Zavanelli	Replace head and deliver by C/S	Would most likely be indicated only if bilateral shoulder dystocia (SD) – anterior shoulder on pubic symphysis and posterior shoulder on sacral promontory.

Post-Delivery

- Neonatal team present for resuscitation
- Take cord gas samples
- Prepare for post-partum haemorrhage – active management of 3rd stage
- Thorough perineal check for trauma, including 3rd and 4th degree tears (particularly if internal manoeuvres were required)
- Thorough documentation including accurate timings
- Debrief of woman, partner and staff

Maternal Collapse/Cardiac Arrest

The cause of maternal collapse may be pregnancy related or non-pregnancy related.

A systematic approach should be used to identify the cause of collapse; potential causes include the 4 Hs and 4 Ts, plus eclampsia and intracranial haemorrhage, plus some additional specific obstetric causes. These are outlined in **Table 9.6**.

Management is shown in **Figures 9.6** and **9.7**.

TABLE 9.6

Potential Causes of Maternal Collapse

Hypoxia	Respiratory – pulmonary embolism (PE), failed intubation, aspiration Heart failure Anaphylaxis Eclampsia/Pre-eclampsia toxaemia (PET) – pulmonary oedema, seizure
Hypovolaemia	Haemorrhage – obstetric (may be concealed), abnormal placentation, uterine rupture, atony, splenic artery/hepatic rupture, aneurysm rupture Cardiac – arrhythmia, myocardial infarction (MI) Distributive – sepsis, high regional block, anaphylaxis
Hypo/hyperkelaemia	Also consider blood sugar, sodium, calcium and magnesium levels
Hypothermia	
Tamponade	Aortic dissection Peripartum cardiomyopathy Trauma
Thrombosis	PE Amniotic fluid embolism (AFE) MI Air embolism
Toxins	Local anaesthetic Magnesium Illicit drugs
Tension pneumothorax	Entonox in pre-existing pneumothorax Trauma

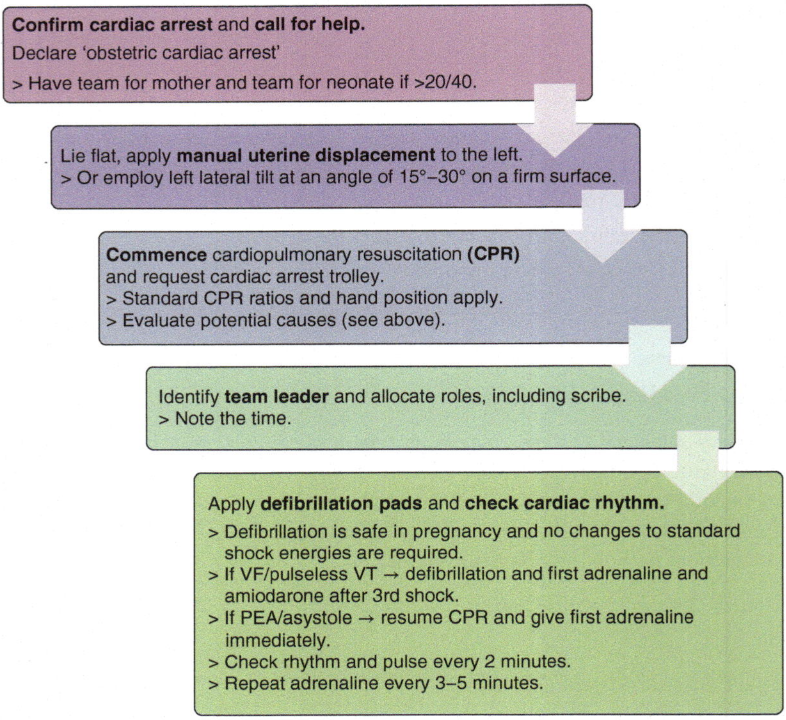

Confirm cardiac arrest and **call for help.**
Declare 'obstetric cardiac arrest'
> Have team for mother and team for neonate if >20/40.

Lie flat, apply **manual uterine displacement** to the left.
> Or employ left lateral tilt at an angle of 15°–30° on a firm surface.

Commence cardiopulmonary resuscitation (**CPR**)
and request cardiac arrest trolley.
> Standard CPR ratios and hand position apply.
> Evaluate potential causes (see above).

Identify **team leader** and allocate roles, including scribe.
> Note the time.

Apply **defibrillation pads** and **check cardiac rhythm.**
> Defibrillation is safe in pregnancy and no changes to standard shock energies are required.
> If VF/pulseless VT → defibrillation and first adrenaline and amiodarone after 3rd shock.
> If PEA/asystole → resume CPR and give first adrenaline immediately.
> Check rhythm and pulse every 2 minutes.
> Repeat adrenaline every 3–5 minutes.

FIGURE 9.6 Management algorithm for maternal cardiac arrest.

Maintain **airway and ventilation.**
> Give 100% oxygen with bag-valve-mask.
> Insert supraglottic airway, or tracheal tube if trained to do so.

Circulation
> Implement IV access above the diaphragm.
> Use IUpper limb intraosseous if IV access unsuccessful.
> Consider extra-corporeal CPR if available.

Emergency **hysterotomy** (perimortem C/S)
> Perform if >20/40, to improve maternal outcome.
> Perform immediately if maternal fatal injuries or prolonged pre-hospital arrest.
> Perform by 5 minutes if no return of spontaneous circulation.

Post resuscitation from **haemorrhage** – active MOH protocol.
> Consider uterotonic drugs, fibrinogen and tranexamic acid (TXA).
> Uterine tamponade/sutures, aortic compression, hysterectomy.

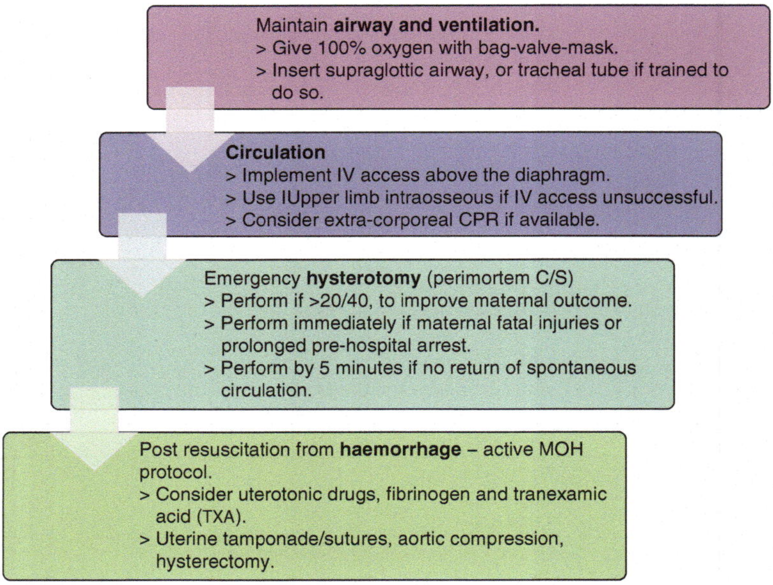

FIGURE 9.7 Management algorithm for maternal cardiac arrest.

Drugs for use during cardiac arrest are shown in **Table 9.7**.

TABLE 9.7

Drugs for Use During Cardiac Arrest

Fluids	**500 mL IV** Crystalloid Bolus
Adrenaline	**1 mg IV** every 3–5 minutes in non-shockable, or after 3rd shock
Amiodarone	**300 mg IV** after 3rd shock
Atropine	**0.5–1 mg IV** up to 3 mg if vagal tone likely cause
Calcium chloride	**10% 10 mL** IV for Mg overdose, low calcium or hyperkalaemia
Magnesium	**2 g IV** for polymorphic VT/hypomagnesaemia **4 g IV** for eclampsia
Thrombolysis/Percutaneous intervention (PCI)	For suspected massive pulmonary embolus/MI
Tranexamic acid	**1 g IV** if haemorrhage
Intralipid	**1.5 mL/kg IV** bolus and **15 mL/kg/hour** IV infusion

Placental Abruption

See **Table 9.8**.

TABLE 9.8

Risk Factors for Placental Abruption

Pre-Existing	**Pregnancy Related**

• Previous abruption
  (*Recurrence risk 4.4% if one previous,*
  up to 25% if two previous)
• Advanced maternal age
• Multiparity
• Low body mass index (BMI)
• Smoking
• Drug misuse
• Maternal thrombophilias
	• Pre-eclampsia
	• Fetal growth restriction
	• Non-vertex presentation
	• Polyhydramnios
	• Assisted reproduction
	• Intrauterine infection
	• prelabour rupture of
	  membranes (PROM)
	• Abdominal trauma
	• First trimester bleeding

Management of Massive Antepartum Haemorrhage (APH) due to Abruption

Perform a rapid assessment to establish whether urgent intervention is required to manage maternal or fetal compromise:

- Is bleeding associated with pain?
- Is uterus tense and woody?
- Assess extent of vaginal bleeding.
- Assess cardiovascular condition of woman.
- Assess fetal well-being.

See Table 9.9 for management of maternal resuscitation and transfusion in the case of massive antepartum haemorrhage.

TABLE 9.9

Steps for Maternal Resuscitation in Case of a Massive Antepartum Haemorrhage

MATERNAL RESUSCITATION
Airway
Assess airway and secure if required.
Breathing
Provide 15 L oxygen via non-rebreathe mask.
Circulation
With two 2 large bore cannulae commence IV fluids. (Until blood is available, transfuse up to 2 L of warmed Hartmanns and/or colloid solution, as rapidly as required.) Send bloods for FBC/U+Es/ X-match/coagulation screen/Kleihauer.
Delivery decision
Assess fetus and decide on delivery.

DELIVERY
• In the event of massive APH, plan and prepare for delivery at the same time as resuscitating the mother.   • Deliver by category 1 C/S.   • Delivery will almost certainly be under general anaesthetic (patient collapsed and hypovolaemic).

BLOOD PRODUCTS
• Aim for X-matched blood if possible.   • If woman is unstable or X-matched blood is unavailable, give type-specific or O-ve blood.   • Cell salvage can be used during C/S, though it is unlikely that time allows to set it up.

Blood product	When to give it	Therapeutic aim
RBC	Empirically in major bleeding	Hb >8 g/dL
FFP 4 units	For every 6 units of red cells Or If PT/APTT >1.5 × control	Prothrombin time <1.5 × mean control APTT <1.5 × mean control
Platelets	Platelet count <50 × 109/L	Platelets >75 × 109/L
Cryoprecipitate	Fibrinogen <1 g/L	Fibrinogen >1 g/L

TABLE 9.9 *(Continued)*

Steps for Maternal Resuscitation in Case of a Massive Antepartum Haemorrhage

POSTNATAL CONSIDERATIONS

- Neonatal team should be present for neonatal resuscitation.
- Prepare for massive post-partum haemorrhage (PPH). Consider the following:
  - Senior obstetrician
  - Additional blood products
  - Additional uterotonics
  - Bakri balloon
  - B-Lynch suture
  - Interventional radiology
  - Hysterectomy
- Consider need for high dependency unit/ intensive care unit (HDU/ITU) care.
- Accurately calculate venous thromboembolism (VTE) risk and appropriate anticoagulation once bleeding risk is low.
- Thoroughly document.
- Debrief of woman, partner and staff.

10

Postnatal Complications

Sepsis

See **Table 10.1**.

TABLE 10.1

Risk Factors for Post-Partum Sepsis

Pre-existing
- Obesity
- Diabetes
- Impaired immunity or immunosuppressive medication
- Anaemia
- History of pelvic infection
- Black or ethnic minority groups

Antenatal
- Amniocentesis/other invasive procedures
- Cervical cerclage
- Prolonged rupture of membranes

Delivery-related
- Vaginal trauma
- Caesarean section
- Wound haematoma
- Retained products of conception

Post-natal
- Vaginal discharge
- GAS infection in close contacts/family members[*]

[*] GAS is increasingly causing invasive infections worldwide.

Assessment

Review of Antenatal History

- Pre-existing risk factors
- Mode of delivery and any complications

 DOI: 10.1201/9781003508151-10

Maternal Assessment

History

- When did she start feeling unwell?
- What systemic symptoms?
  - Fever
  - Rigors
  - Rash
  - Lethargy
  - Reduced appetite
- Local symptoms suggestive of source?
  - Diarrhoea and vomiting (D+V)
  - Breast redness/tenderness/heat
  - Abdo/pelvic pain
  - Wound redness/discharge
  - Offensive vaginal discharge
  - Heavy lochia
  - Productive cough
  - Urinary symptoms
  - Upper respiratory tract symptoms
- Unwell contacts?

Table 10.2 specifies treatment in the case of Group A Streptococcus infection.

TABLE 10.2

Group A Streptococcus

- Hx of Group A Streptococcus (GAS) infection in close contacts?
- Baby should be examined by a paediatrician as neonates are especially susceptible to streptococcal and staphylococcal infections.
- Other household contacts should be counselled about symptoms of GAS, and some may need prophylaxis.
- GAS identified during pregnancy or the puerperium should be treated aggressively.

Maternal Observations

- Plot on MEWS chart.
- Perform Sepsis 6 if triggered by observations.

Examination

Top-to-toe assessment (specific examinations depend on any local symptoms reported)

- Upper respiratory tract – tonsillar exudate, lymphadenopathy
- Breast examination – engorgement, redness, tenderness, heat, discharge

- Abdominal palpation – involution of uterus, tenderness of uterus, signs of wound infection (if delivery by lower section caesarean section [LSCS])
- Perineal examination (if trauma) – swelling, redness, tenderness, discharge, haematoma
- Soft tissue changes at site of previous cannulae/injections/spinals
- Lower limbs – signs of thrombosis (red, tender, swollen)

Speculum examination

- Assess lochia (amount, colour, smell)
- High vaginal swab (HVS) for MC+S

Investigations (depending on signs and symptoms)

- Full observations[*a]
- Full blood count (FBC), Urea and electrolytes (U+Es), liver function tests (LFTs), coagulation screen
- Arterial blood gas ABG/VBG if clinically unwell
- Bacterial/Viral throat swabs
- Sputum
- Swabs of any breast discharge/breast milk
- HVS/low vaginal swab (LVS)
- Urine for M,C+S
- Epidural site swab/cerebro-spinal fluid (CSF) (if epidural site is suspected source)
- Stool sample if diarrhoea
- Placenta swabs (if immediately postnatal)

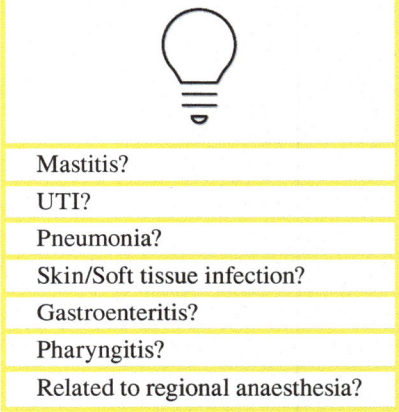

| Mastitis? |
| UTI? |
| Pneumonia? |
| Skin/Soft tissue infection? |
| Gastroenteritis? |
| Pharyngitis? |
| Related to regional anaesthesia? |

[*a] The following clinical signs are suggestive of sepsis:

- Pyrexia
- Hypothermia
- Tachycardia
- Tachypnoea
- Hypoxia
- Hypotension
- Oliguria
- Impaired consciousness
- Failure to respond to treatment

(Use thresholds according to local modified early obstetric warning score [MEOWS] chart in use.)

Imaging (depending on suspected site of infection)

- Chest X-ray
- Pelvic ultrasound scan (USS)
- Computed tomography (CT) abdo-pelvis

Management of Postnatal Sepsis (Tables 10.3, 10.4 and Figure 10.1)

- Patients with suspected post-partum sepsis should be managed in hospital with an high-dependency unit/intensive care unit (HDU/ITU).
- Patients should be isolated and all health care workers should wear appropriate personal protective equipment (PPE).
- Prompt initiation of Sepsis 6 bundle (**Table 10.3**) is paramount in the management of post-partum sepsis.
- Local guidance should be followed with regards to the most appropriate antibiotic treatment, with relevant consideration of
  - Likely focus of infection
  - Likely causative microorganism
  - Safety of antibiotic in breastfeeding women
  - Local resistance profiles
- Seek and treat the focus of infection:
  - Uterine evacuation if retained products of conception (RPOC) and endometritis
  - Drainage of abscess/haematoma (pelvic/perineal/breast/wound)
- Close liaison with the MDT.
- Involve critical care outreach team to consider transfer to high dependency or intensive care unit (**Table 10.4** for indications for transfer).

TABLE 10.3

Sepsis Six Bundle

1. Give oxygen (maintain sats >94%).
2. Take blood cultures.
3. Give IV antibiotics.
4. Give IV fluid challenge.
5. Measure lactate.
6. Measure urine output.

TABLE 10.4

Indication for Transfer to ITU

System	Indication
Cardiovascular	Hypotension Raised serum lactate (>4) despite fluid resuscitation
Respiratory	Pulmonary oedema Mechanical ventilation Airway protection
Renal	Renal dialysis
Neurological	Significantly decreased conscious level
Miscellaneous	Multiorgan failure Uncorrected acidosis Hypothermia

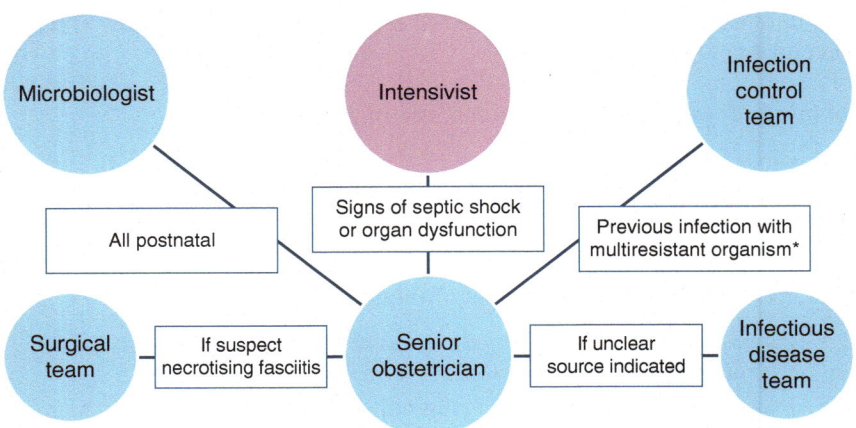

FIGURE 10.1 Potential management colleagues. *Note*: *Extended-spectrum beta lactamase (ESBL)-producing organisms, methicillin-resistant *Staphylococcus aureus* (MRSA), GAS, Panton-Valentine leukocidin (PVL)-producing *Staphylococci*.

Anaemia (Table 10.5)

For the acute management of post-partum haemorrhage, please refer to Chapter 3.

TABLE 10.5

Risk Factors for Post-Partum Anaemia

Pre-existing
- Pre-existing anaemia
- Haemoglobinopathies

Antenatal
- Uncorrected antenatal anaemia
- Uncorrected B12/Ferritin deficiencies

Delivery-related
- Post-partum haemorrhage
- Vaginal trauma
- Operative vaginal delivery
- Caesarean section (C/S)
- Wound haematoma
- Retained products of conception

Postnatal
- Secondary post-partum haemorrhage (PPH)
- Excessive lochia

Assessment

1. **Review of antenatal history**
   - Pre-existing risk factors
   - Mode of delivery and any complications
   - Any treatment of anaemia to date (including blood transfusion)
2. **Maternal assessment**

History

- General well-being
  - Has patient mobilised since delivery? Any symptoms (Sx) of anaemia (light headed, shortness of breath (SOB), palpitations)?
  - Feeling particularly fatigued (although difficult to distinguish from normal post-partum fatigue)?
- Per vaginal (PV) bleeding
  - How often is patient needing to change her pads?
  - Any change in colour/smell of PV loss?
- Pain
  - Abdominal pain of severity that does not fit with mode of delivery should warrant further investigation.

Examination

- Perform a full set of observations and document on a MEOWS chart.
- General appearance – pallor, mucous membranes, mobilising effectively?
- Abdominal examination – palpate uterus for involution, tone, tenderness.
- Assess PV loss – if appears excessive on pad, or if concerns with uterine examination, then perform speculum examination to assess for excessive loss/clots/signs of infection.
- Perineum – assess blood loss from any perineal trauma and examine to rule out a haematoma.

Investigations

- Bloods – FBC, coagulation, group and save (G+S)
- ABG for Hb if patient appears acutely unwell

Imaging

- Consider pelvic/abdominal USS if you suspect bleeding/endometritis secondary to retained products of conception.
- Perform CT abdo-pelvis if Hb dropping with minimal visible blood loss – may indicate pelvic haematoma/intra-abdominal bleed (particularly, but not exclusively, following C/S).

Management

Rule out any source of ongoing bleeding as a priority.

 Always consider infection/sepsis as a cause of anaemia in the puerperium.

Oral Iron Replacement

- In patients with Hb <105 who are clinically stable, oral iron replacement therapy can be offered.
- See **Table 10.6** for options of medication regimes.
- Patients should be advised to take iron tablets on an empty stomach. Taking with a source of Vitamin C (e.g. orange juice) will enhance absorption, and tea/coffee should be avoided for an hour after taking iron tablets as absorption is limited by tannins.

TABLE 10.6

Preparations for Iron Salts

Iron salt	Preparation
Ferrous fumarate	210 mg
Ferrous gluconate	300 mg
Ferrous sulphate (dried)	200 mg
Ferrous feredate	190 mg/5 mL elixir

Note: Once-daily dosing or alternate-day dosing is optimum to increase absorption.

- Watch for potential side effects: gastrointestinal (GI) effects, constipation.
- Will restore Hb but prolonged course likely to be needed. Ferritin levels likely to increase, but to a lesser extent than if IV iron were used.

IV Iron Replacement

- In patients with Hb <105 who are clinically stable, IV iron therapy can be offered as an alternative to oral iron.
- Benefits include quicker restoration of Hb and better and sustained improvement in ferritin levels.
- Risks include small chance of medication reaction (very rare), risk of permanent skin staining if iron leaks into tissues (e.g. if cannula not inserted correctly).

Blood Transfusion

- In patients with Hb <70, and/or symptomatic of anaemia, blood transfusion can be offered on an individualised basis.
- Benefits include immediate replacement of oxygen-carrying capacity of blood and thus improvement in symptoms.
- Risks include transfusion reactions, infections, less sustained improvement in Hb levels.

Perineal Trauma

See **Table 10.7**.

TABLE 10.7

Risk Factors for Perineal Trauma

Pre-existing
- Perineal scarring
- Previous 3rd or 4th degree tear

Antenatal
- Primip
- Large for gestational age baby
- No perineal massage performed

Delivery-related
- Prolonged labour
- Instrumental delivery
- No hands on/warm compress/perineal support during second stage
- Need for episiotomy

Assessment

1. **Review of delivery and perineal trauma**
   - Mode of delivery, degree of perineal trauma sustained, type of repair
   - Plan from person repairing trauma (e.g. need for antibiotics/laxatives)
2. **Maternal assessment**

History

- Perineal pain and what analgesics are being used?
- Has patient passed urine? Bowels opened?

Examination

- Perform a full set of observations and document on a MEOWS chart.
- General appearance – any signs of anaemia or infection?
- Perineum – assess trauma – swelling, erythema, discharge. Ensure no signs of haematoma (exquisitely tender firm red/purple lump in perineum indicates haematoma).

Investigations

- Bloods for anaemia/infection if any concerns.

Advice

- General advice following any perineal trauma
  - Pain – treat with paracetamol, ibuprofen, cold compress. May require codeine for first one to two days.
  - Hygiene – pour warm water over perineum to rinse after toileting; wipe front to back after opening bowels. Pat area dry rather than rubbing to avoid disturbing stitches.
  - Bowel opening – gentle pressure with clean pad over trauma can make this more comfortable; good hydration and high fibre diet help to reduce constipation (laxatives may be required).
  - Signs of infection – observe for redness, swelling, discharge from trauma, offensive smell, persistent pain.
  - Pelvic floor exercise – start as soon as comfortable to enhance healing and reduce scar tissue.
- Following 3rd of fourth degree perineal tear
  - Prescribe antibiotics to reduce risk of infection.
  - Provide laxatives to avoid constipation; also advise good hydration and high-fibre diet.
  - Refer to obstetric anal sphincter injury (OASI) clinic for three-month follow up.
  - Refer to physio for pelvic floor exercise.
  - Next pregnancy will need discussion re mode of delivery depending on ongoing symptoms and patient preference.

Postnatal urinary retention

Risk Factors

- Instrumental delivery
- Epidural analgesia
- Episiotomy
- Nulliparity

Prolonged use of Syntocinon and excessive use of opioids are also linked to voiding problems postnatally.

Suggested Management

See **Figure 10.2**.
Following insertion of an indwelling catheter

- The patient should be advised to keep a record of their fluid intake for the first 4 hours after insertion.
- Antibiotics should be considered.

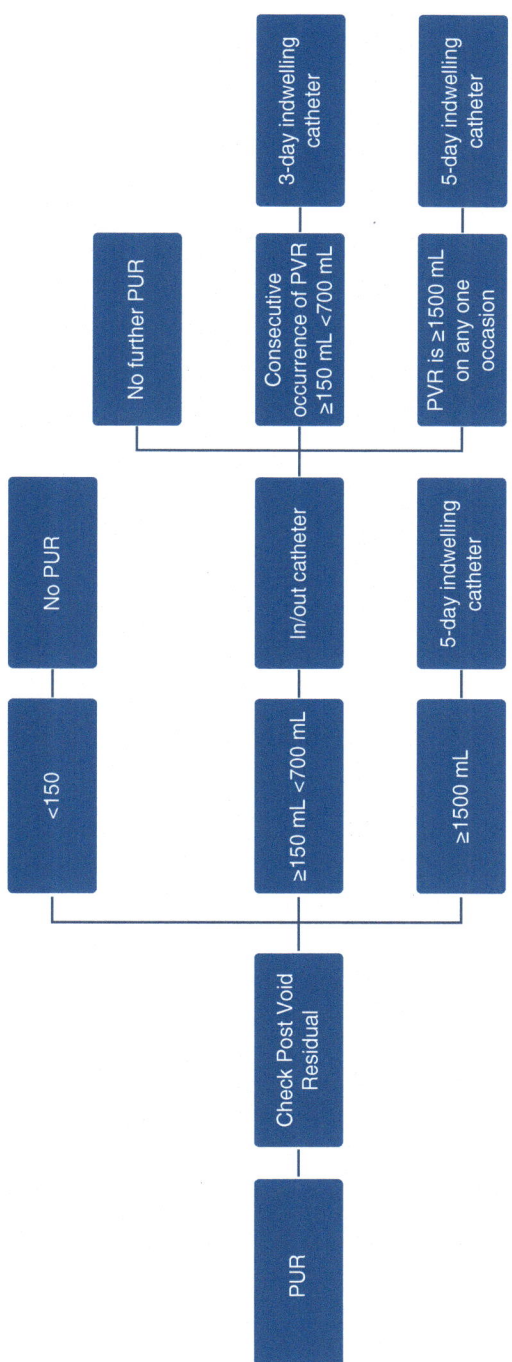

FIGURE 10.2 Management algorithm for postnatal urinary retention (PUR).

11

Summaries

TABLE 11.1

Advanced Maternal Age (>40)

Antenatal	Extra tests	• Emphasise importance of screening due to higher risk of chromosomal abnormalities. • Increased chance of pre-existing medical conditions – optimise management and medications. • Increased risk pre-eclamptic toxaemia (PET)/gestational diabetes mellitus (GDM) but no role for routine screening.
	Extra scans	• Advanced age alone not an indication for serial scans.
	Delivery	• Advanced age alone not indication for LSCS, but many older mothers may choose this – discuss individually depending on circumstances. • Induction of labour (IOL) from 39/40 (women age >40 have similar stillbirth risk at 39/40 compared to 25–29-year-olds at 41/40).
Intrapartum	Increased risk/prophylaxis for increased risk	• There is increased rate of lower section caesarean section (LSCS) for labour dystocia and increased rate of instrumental delivery. • During IOL, women more likely to need Syntocinon at higher doses and for longer to achieve successful vaginal delivery.
	Monitoring in labour	• No indication for cEFM unless other comorbidities.
Postnatal		• Increased risk PPH – advise active management of third stage.
Future pregnancies		• Risks discussed here will increase with advancing maternal age.
Counselling points		• At 41/40, stillbirth (SB) risk is 0.75:1000 for women <35y, but 2.5:1000 for women ≥40 year. (This effect persists after accounting for medical disease, parity, race and ethnicity). • IOL at 39/40 aims to reduce late antenatal stillbirths and maternal risks of an ongoing pregnancy such as pre-eclampsia (PET). • IOL at 39 weeks does not seem to increase number of instrumental or caesarean deliveries.

DOI: 10.1201/9781003508151-11

TABLE 11.2

Raised BMI (≥30)

Antenatal	Extra tests	• High dose folic acid (5 mg OD) until 12/40 • Vitamin D supplementation • Risk of GDM – for glucose tolerance test (GTT) at 26–28/40 • Risk pregnancy-induced hypertension (PIH)/PET – no additional monitoring indicated, but ensure correct BP cuff size used • Re-weigh at 36/40 • Appropriate assessments for aspirin and thromboprophylaxis • Dietician review **In addition, for women with BMI ≥40:** • Antenatal assessment by obstetric anaesthetist (multi-disciplinary team [MDT] involvement where significant potential difficulties are identified) • Moving and handling risk assessment in 3rd trimester
	Extra scans	• Serial growth scans for BMI ≥35
	Delivery	• Can consider IOL at term to lower chance of needing LSCS
Intrapartum	Increased risk/prophylaxis for increased risk	• Can be midwifery-led care [MLC] if multip with no other risk factors and BMI <40. (Individual units likely to have their own policy on this.) • If body mass index (BMI) ≥40, advise consultant led care (CLC) and inform on-call anaesthetist when admitted in labour. • If BMI ≥40, early IV access in labour (plus consider second cannula). • If having LSCS, increased risk of wound infection – prophylactic abx, suture fat layer, consider surgical drain and negative pressure dressing.
	Monitoring in labour	• Raised BMI alone not an indication for continuous external fetal monitoring (cEFM).
Postnatal		• Risk of post-partum haemorrhage (PPH) – active management of third stage and consider 40 units Syntocinon prophylactically. • Breastfeeding support as rates are lower in women with raised BMI.
Future pregnancies		• Weight loss between pregnancies lowers risk of SB, hypertensive complications and fetal macrosomia, and improves chance of successful vaginal birth after caesarean (VBAC).
Counselling points		• Raised BMI increases complications in the antenatal (gestational diabetes mellitus [GDM], PET, macrosomia, small for gestational age [SGA]), intrapartum (difficulty monitoring, labour dystocia, ↑risk LSCS) and postpartum (PPH, infection, difficulty with breastfeeding) periods. • Weight loss prior to and between pregnancies will reduce these risks, in a linear fashion.

TABLE 11.3

Low BMI (<18.5)

Antenatal	Extra tests	• Screen for underlying eating disorders
		  • Refer to specialist in eating disorders (ED), and dietician if co-existing condition present.
		  • Establish if there is use of appetite suppressants, laxatives or diuretics.
		• Test full blood count (FBC), urea and electrolytes (U+Es), liver function tests (LFTs), bone profile, vitamin D.
		• If low Hb – ferritin, B12, folate (and treat anaemia and other deficiencies).
		• Perform urinalysis – ketonuria may suggest forced emesis/starvation.
		• Consider if any safeguarding concerns.

	Extra scans	• Do serial ultrasound scan (USS) if BMI <18 (or if <20 with another risk factor for growth restriction). • Also consider in those with poor weight gain in pregnancy.
	Delivery	• Early delivery indicated only if concerns with fetal growth. • Be aware that tokophobia is more common amongst this group of women.

Intrapartum	Increased risk/prophylaxis for increased risk	• Increased risk of late preterm delivery 34–37/40
		  • Consider steroids if <36/40
		  • MgSO$_4$ if <34/40

	Monitoring in labour	• Only if concerns with fetal growth
Postnatal		• Ongoing care by dietician if required • Bone density scan if indicated
Future pregnancies		• Aim for BMI in normal range for future pregnancies. • If eating disorder present, aim for this to be in remission prior to future pregnancies.
Counselling points		• Low BMI is protective against many complications including PIH, PET, GDM, large for gestational age (LFGA), need for LSCS.

TABLE 11.4

Smokers

Antenatal	Extra tests	• CO level at booking and then at every antenatal visit • Considered a 'smoker' if smoked cigarettes at time of, or any time since conception. • Vaping/e-cigarette use not counted as a smoker. • Refer to smoking cessation service
	Extra scans	• Serial USS from 28/40 if smoker of ≥10/day (or if CO reading >4 ppm)
	Delivery	• No indication for early delivery if growth normal
Intrapartum	Increased risk/prophylaxis for increased risk	• Nil additional if no growth concerns antenatally
	Monitoring in labour	• Only if small for gestational age or other fetal concerns
Postnatal		• Postnatal -refer to smoking cessation services if patient consents, and emphasise importance of stopping smoking with regards to maternal health, and also reducing risk of neonatal mortality
Future pregnancies		• Aim for patient to be smoke-free at time of conception of next pregnancy to avoid associated risks
Counselling points		• Smoking is associated with ↑risk of miscarriage, stillbirth, abruption, preterm birth and low birth weight.

TABLE 11.5

Varicella Zoster Virus (VZV/Chickenpox)

Antenatal	Extra tests	• If a pregnant woman has had contact with chickenpox, see appendix for algorithm. • If chickenpox rash develops, woman should see GP and avoid contact with susceptible individuals, including other pregnant women and babies, until lesions have crusted over. • If >20/40 and present within 24 h of onset of rash, treat with acyclovir **800mg five times daily for seven days.** • If signs and symptoms of severe chickenpox (respiratory symptoms, photophobia, seizures, drowsiness haemorrhagic rash/bleeding, dense rash), inpatient management is required by MDT; IV acyclovir will be required.
	Extra scans	• Fetal medicine scan at 16–20 weeks, or 5 weeks after infection
	Delivery	• Planned delivery should be delayed for at least 7 days after onset of rash wherever possible.

Intrapartum	Increased risk/prophylaxis for increased risk	• Delivery whilst vesicles are active may be extremely hazardous
		  • May precipitate haemorrhage/coagulopathy due to thrombocytopenia/hepatitis.
		  • High risk of varicella in newborn – significant morbidity and mortality.
		• If active chickenpox at time of delivery.
		  • IV acyclovir
		  • Epidural/spinal site free of cutaneous lesions
		  • Care in isolation – avoid contact with other pregnant women/babies/non-immune staff

	Monitoring in labour	
Postnatal		• Inform neonatal team if baby born to mother who developed chicken pox at any stage in pregnancy. • Babies born to mothers who have chickenpox rash from 7 days prior to 7 days after delivery should receive VZIG +/– acyclovir. • No contraindication to breastfeeding.
Future pregnancies		• Postnatal vaccination should be advised to all non-immune women to ensure immunity in subsequent pregnancies (no contraindication to breastfeeding after receiving vaccine postnatally).
Counselling points		• VZV <28/40 – risk of fetal varicella syndrome post-exposure prophylaxis in susceptible pregnant women reduces risk of developing FVS). • VZV in last 4 weeks of pregnancy – significant risk of varicella infection in newborn.

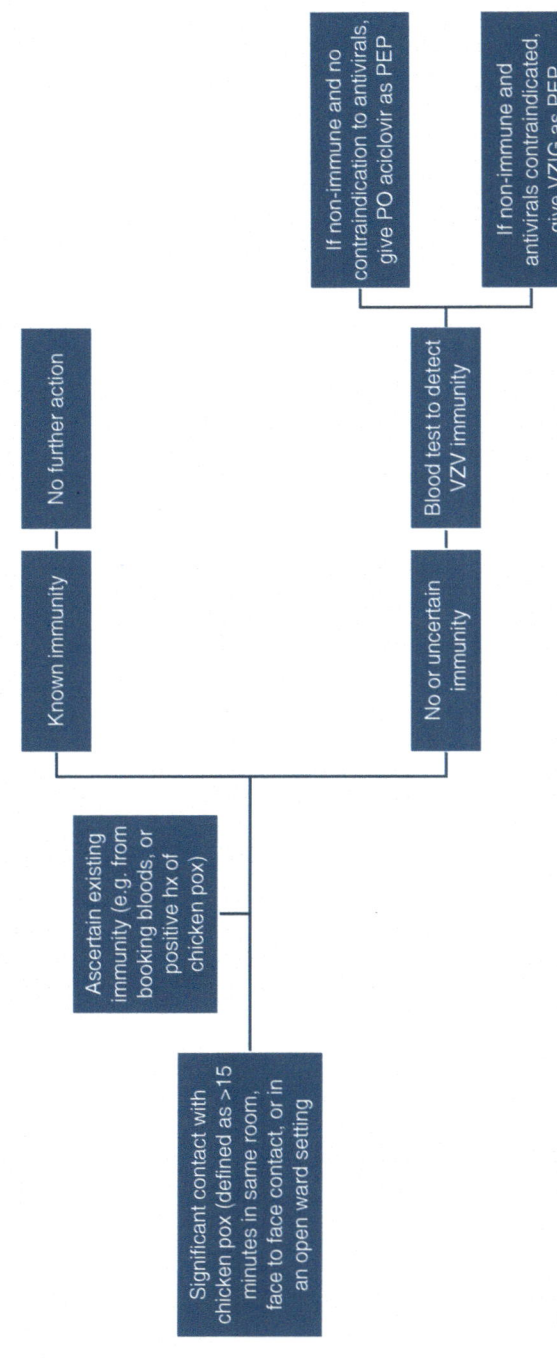

FIGURE 11.1   Algorithm for the management of VZV exposure in pregnancy.

TABLE 11.6

Genital Herpes in Pregnancy – Primary Infection

Antenatal	Extra tests	Acquisition <28/40 • Refer to genitourinary medicine (GUM) to confirm diagnosis. • Commence acyclovir 400 mg three times a day (TDS) for 5/7 (do not delay starting whilst awaiting Dx). • IV acyclovir for disseminated herpes • If delivery doesn't occur within 6 weeks, then prepare expectant management and plan vaginal delivery. • Give acyclovir 400mg TDS from 36/40 to reduce herpes lesions at term. Acquisition ≥28/40 • Check antibody status to confirm this is first episode of infection. • Commence acyclovir 400mg TDS and continue as suppression until delivery. • Advise delivery by elective LSCS (if symptoms within 6w of delivery, risk of neonatal transmission = 41%). Preterm prelabour rupture of membranes (PPROM) • MDT discussion re timing of delivery – limited evidence • If initial conservative Mx – IV acyclovir 5 mg/kg 8 hourly • Steroids as per usual protocol • Benefit of LSCS delivery within 6 weeks of primary infection, even with PPROM
	Extra scans	None indicated
	Delivery	• LSCS if primary infection acquired in third trimester • LSCS if herpes lesions noted at onset of labour and no prior h/o herpes infection
Intrapartum	Increased risk/prophylaxis for increased risk	• If woman opting for vaginal delivery, give IV acyclovir 5 mg/kg 8-hourly (and then to baby). • For those who deliver vaginally in presence of active lesions, avoid invasive procedures such as fetal scalp electrode (FSE)/fetal blood sampling (FBS)/ artificial rupture of membranes (ARM)/instrumental delivery.
	Monitoring in labour	Nil additional
Postnatal		• Inform neonatal team. • Conservative MX if born by LSCS • IF spontaneous vaginal delivery (SVD) (with active lesions/within 6/52 of primary infection) – herpes simplex virus polymerase (HSV PCR) swabs and empirical Rx with IV acyclovir • Breastfeeding recommended unless herpetic lesions around nipples.

(Continued)

TABLE 11.6 *(Continued)*

Genital Herpes in Pregnancy – Primary Infection

Future pregnancies	• As per table outlining management of recurrent HSV infection
Counselling points	• Rx with acyclovir reduces duration and severity of symptoms and duration of viral shedding. • Aciclovir is unlicensed in pregnancy, but no maternal/neonatal adverse outcomes reported. • Risk of neonatal transmission is highest if infection has been acquired within six weeks of delivery, as seroconversion has not completed. Risk is up to 41%.

TABLE 11.7

Genital Herpes in Pregnancy – Recurrent Infection

Antenatal	Extra tests	• Most episodes are short-lasting and self-resolve in seven to ten days without antiviral treatment. • Supportive treatment – paracetamol, saline bathing, topical lidocaine gel. • Suppressive acyclovir 400 mg TDS PO (reduces viral shedding and recurrence at delivery, thus need for LSCS. NO effect on transmission rates.) PPROM • <34/40 – expectant management with PO acyclovir 400 mg TDS • >34/40 – manage as per PPROM guidance
	Extra scans	• Not indicated
	Delivery	• Plan for SVD (unless other obstetric indications for LSCS).
Intrapartum	Increased risk/prophylaxis for increased risk	• If lesions present at onset of delivery in a recurrent infection, transmission rate remains low at 0%–3% and so vaginal delivery should be encouraged. • If SROM at term, expedite delivery to minimise duration of fetal exposure to HSV.
	Monitoring in labour	• Nil additional for HSV
Postnatal		• Inform neonatal team. • Conservative management advised (unless concerns with the neonate, e.g. sepsis/poor feeding).
Future pregnancies		• Risk of transmission will remain low at 0%–3% for recurrences in future pregnancies.
Counselling points		• In recurrent infection, risk of neonatal transmission is low at 0%–3%, even if lesions present at time of delivery.

TABLE 11.8

Human Immunodeficiency Virus (HIV)

Antenatal	Extra tests	*Note that individual assisted reproductive techniques (ART) and combined anti-retroviral therapy (cART) regimes are not outlined here due to their complexity – please refer to the British HIV Association (BHIVA) guideline on HIV in pregnancy for full details.*
		
		• Sexual health screening should be performed for all women with HIV, whether pre-existing or newly diagnosed in pregnancy.
		• For women conceiving on cART, there should be a minimum of one CD4 cell count at baseline and one at delivery.
		• For women commencing cART in pregnancy, an HIV viral load should be performed 2–4 weeks after starting cART, at least once each trimester, at 36/40 and at delivery.
		• All pregnant women, including elite controllers, should start ART during pregnancy and be advised to continue life-long treatment.
		• For women not on cART, commence cART
		  • As soon as able in 2nd trimester if baseline viral load <30,000 HIV RNA copies/mL
		  • At start of 2nd trimester if baseline viral load 30,000 – 100,000 HIV RNA copies/mL
		  • In 1st trimester if viral load >100,000 HIV RNAA copies/mL, or CD4 count <200cells/mm^3
		• Combined screening and non-invasive pre-natal testing (NIPT) for those who are high risk will reduce number of women needing invasive testing. (If invasive testing is required it should be performed when viral load <50 HIV RNA copies/mL.).
		• ECV can be offered to women with plasma viral load <50 HIV RNA copies/mL.

	Extra scans	• Nil additional scans unless other obstetric indications
	Delivery	• Advise vaginal delivery if viral load <50 at 36/40. • If viral load 50–399 at 36/40, consider el LSCS depending on trajectory of viral load, length of time on treatment, adherence issues, obstetric issues and the woman's views. • If viral load ≥400 at 36/40, elective LSCS is recommended at 38–39/40.
Intrapartum	Increased risk/prophylaxis for increased risk	• If pre-labour spontaneous rupture of membranes (SROM), aim to deliver within 24 hours of SROM. (I.e. offer immediate IOL/LSCS depending on viral load at 36/40, as above.) • If SROM ≥34/40, follow above guidance, with addition of GBS prophylaxis. • If SROM <34/40; steroids for fetal lung maturation, optimise viral load, MDT discussion re timing and mode of delivery.
	Monitoring in labour	• As per other obstetric indications
Postnatal		• Post-exposure prophylaxis (PEP) for baby as per guidance; advise against breast feeding. • Advise woman to continue cART postpartum. Discuss and offer contraception. • Cervical smear three months post-delivery.

TABLE 11.9

Hepatitis B (HBV)

Antenatal	Extra tests	• Women should be managed by MDT with involvement of obstetrician, specialist midwife, virologist. • Women with known HBV should have HBV serology and HBV DNA sent for testing at booking to allow infectivity status to be assessed. • Women on antiviral treatment for HBV prior to pregnancy should continue treatment during and after pregnancy. • Women with confirmed HBV should also be offered screening for HIV/HCV and hepatitis delta. • If HBV DNA >200,000 IU/mL, or quantitative HBsAg >4 log10 IU/mL, offer antiviral treatment from 24/40. (Tenofovir disoproxil is the preferred choice of antiviral treatment during pregnancy.) • Assess for liver disease – bloods (FBC, U+Es, LFTs, clotting) and liver USS in first trimester. • If raised ALT in pregnancy, test HBV DNA to rule out a viral flare. • In women with cirrhosis, morbidity and mortality are high. Manage in conjunction with specialist hepatology centre.
	Extra scans	• Nil additional required. • Note that antenatal invasive procedures can be performed in women with HBV infection. (In women with a high viral load, small risk of HBV transmission should be balanced against benefit of antenatal invasive testing.)
Intrapartum	Delivery	• HBV is not an indication for LSCS.
	Increased risk/prophylaxis for increased risk	• Avoid invasive procedures (FSE/FBS/difficult instrumentals) to reduce risk of vertical transmission.
	Monitoring in labour	• Nil additional in HBV infection.
Postnatal		• Women on antiviral therapy for prevention of HBV vertical transmission should stop by 12/52 post-partum. • Can breastfeed as long as baby immunised within 24 hours of birth, and no co-infection with HIV.
Future pregnancies		• HBV DNA will need to be tested at booking in all future pregnancies to determine infectivity status. • Women on antiviral treatment should be advised to continue this if they conceive in future.
Counselling points		• In women who are newly diagnosed with HBV, household and contact screening should be advised. • Risk of transmission is 70%–90% from a hepatitis B e-antigen positive mother, and 10%–40% in a hepatitis B e-antigen negative mother without prophylaxis. Antiviral therapy reduces this risk significantly.

TABLE 11.10

Previous Hypertensive Disease

Antenatal	Extra tests	• Baseline U+Es if pre-existing hypertension.
		• Optimise medications (labetalol/nifedipine first line, methyldopa can be used but risk PN depression so should be stopped after birth).
		• Aspirin 150 mg ON from 12/40
		  • Closely monitor of BP and urinalysis throughout pregnancy:
		    • Weekly if BP poorly controlled
		• 2–4 weekly if well controlled
		• sFlt:PLGF ratio if suspicion of developing PET.

	Extra scans	• Serial growth scans if previous severe PET/preterm birth (PTB) <34/40 due to PET/previous PET with SGA <10th centile/previous abruption
	Delivery	• No indication for early delivery if index pregnancy is uncomplicated. • IOL from 37/40 if on medication for pre-existing hypertension, depending on BP control
Intrapartum	Increased risk/prophylaxis for increased risk	• Risk of developing intrapartum hypertension/PET • Regular BP monitoring in labour and act accordingly if concerns
	Monitoring in labour	Only if BP concerns this pregnancy.

Postnatal		• Additional BP monitoring if on medication for chronic hypertension
		  • Daily for two days, once between days three to five
		  • Continue anti-hypertensive (but change if on methyldopa), aim BP <140/90 (omit medication if BP <110/70)
		  • R/v of medication two weeks post-natal
		• Risk hypertension/PET in first 48 hours following delivery

Future pregnancies		• Monitoring/prophylaxis as per this pregnancy as risk recurrence remains

TABLE 11.11

Hypertensive Disease of Pregnancy – Pregnancy-Induced Hypertension and Pre-Eclampsia

Antenatal	Extra tests	• Regular BP monitoring (depending on severity of hypertension). Urine dip for proteinuria, and urinary protein:creatinine ratio. Bloods for FBC, U+Es, LFTs, Coagulation screen, Sflt:plGF ratio of available locally • Hospitalisation if sustained BP ≥160 mmHg, ↑creatinine, ↑ALT, ↓platelets, signs of impending eclampsia or CTG concerns
	Extra scans	• Serial USS for EFW and UAD once PIH/PET diagnosed (2–4 weekly depending on severity of PET and scan findings)
	Delivery	• 37–40/40 for PIH depending on medication and control of BP • 37/40 for PET, earlier if maternal/fetal concerns (discuss with consultant)

Intrapartum	Increased risk/prophylaxis for increased risk	• Risk of prematurity in planned early birth:
		  • Consider steroids <35+6/40
		  • MgSO₄ <34/40
		• Risk of worsening htn / progression to/of PET:
		  • Hourly BP monitoring, or every 15 minutes if BP >160/110
		  • Continue anti-hypertensives during labour
		  • Bloods for platelets, U+Es, LFTs if worsening of BP/proteinuria/symptoms
		  • Fluid restriction to 80 mL/hour in severe PET
		  • MgSO₄ for eclampsia prevention if BP uncontrollable, worsening symptoms or worsening bloods.

	Monitoring in labour	Continuous external fetal monitoring (cEFM)

Postnatal		• For PIH
		  • Continue anti-hypertensive treatment (except methyldopa – stop by day two)
		  • BP daily for two days, once between days three to five
		  • Review of BP and medication at two weeks postnatal
		• For PET
		  • Continue anti-hypertensive treatment (except methyldopa – stop by day two)
		  • Bloods for platelets, U+Es and LFTs 48–72 h after birth
		  • BP 4x daily whilst inpatient and then every one or two days for up to two weeks until no medication and BP normal

Future pregnancies		• See table of management for women with previous hypertensive disease.

TABLE 11.12

Intrahepatic Cholestasis of Pregnancy (ICP; Commonly Known as Obstetric Cholestasis)

Antenatal	Extra tests	• Consider if woman presents with itching with no skin changes.
		• Repeat LFTs and BAs 2–weekly if normal but itching persists.
		• Bile acid level >19 µmol/L supports dx of ICP.
		  • mild; 19–39
		  • moderate; 40–99
		  • severe; ≥100
		• Weekly BAs to help plan timing of birth
		• Emollients/antihistamines for symptomatic control of itch
		• No role for UDCA in reducing BAs/improving pregnancy outcome.
		• Perform viral/autoimmune screen only if other LFTs are markedly abnormal.
		• ↑risk PET – perform regular BP and urine check.
		• Essential for woman to present if concerns with altered fetal movements.

	Extra scans	• USS does not predict SB in IHP. • Fetal death occurs despite normal EFW/Doppler studies.
	Delivery	• Routine care in mild IHP • 38–39 weeks in moderate IHP • 35–36 weeks in severe IHP (If presence of co-morbidities such as gestational diabetes mellitus (GDM) or PET, multiple pregnancy should lower threshold for earlier planned delivery.)

Intrapartum	Increased risk/prophylaxis for increased risk	• ↑risk PTB in moderate/severe ICP (spontaneous or iatrogenic)
		  • Steroids if planning early delivery/patient presents in TPTL <36/60
		  • MgSO₄ if planning earlier delivery/patient presents in TPTL <34/40
		• ↑risk meconium-stained liquor in moderate/severe ICP

	Monitoring in labour	• cEFM if BAs ≥100 µmol/L, and/or in presence of meconium
Postnatal		• ↑chance neonatal intensive care unit (NICU) admission – paediatrician at birth. • Check LFTs and BAs no sooner than four weeks after birth to ensure resolution. If not resolved, consider a cause other than/in addition to ICP.
Future pregnancies		• Increased risk of recurrence of IHP in future pregnancies • Baseline liver function tests (LFTs) and bile acids (BAs) with booking bloods in next pregnancy.
Counselling points		• Stillbirth rate increased above baseline risk only if BA concentration ≥100 µmol/L. • Stillbirth rate similar to background risk until 38–39/40 if BA concentration 40–99 µmol/L. • Stillbirth rate unchanged for all gestations if BA concentration 19–39 µmol/L.

TABLE 11.13

Gestational Diabetes (GDM)

Antenatal	Extra tests	• *Indications for GTT*: BMI >30, previous baby >4.5kg, previous GDM, 1st degree relative with diabetes, ethnicity with high prevalence of diabetes, significant glycosuria (2+ on 1 occasion or 1+ on 2 occasions)
		• After diagnosis, see in joint diabetic ANC within one week (and then 1–2 weekly)
		  • If fasting BG <7 at diagnosis, offer dietary and exercise changes. If targets not met within 1 week, offer metformin, then add insulin if required.
		  • If fasting BG >7 at diagnosis, offer insulin +/– metformin.
		• Refer to dietician.

	Extra scans	• Serial USS for estimated fetal weight (EFW) and umbilical artery doppler (UAD).
	Delivery	• By 40+6/40 if no complications
Intrapartum	Increased risk/prophylaxis for increased risk	• Blood sugar (BM) monitoring hourly during labour and for sliding scale if BMs not controlled between 4 and 7 mmol/L. • Increased risk of shoulder dystocia, especially if macrosomic fetus (increased fat deposition between shoulder blades in fetus to mother with diabetes) – be aware of slow progress/high station.
	Monitoring in labour	• cEFM advised in all except diet– controlled GDM.
Postnatal		• Stop all glucose-lowering therapy immediately after birth. • Fasting glucose or HbA1c 6–3 weeks postnatal to exclude diabetes • Annual Hb1Ac thereafter
Future pregnancies		• Risk recurrence in future pregnancies – for GTT ASAP after booking, and then repeated at 24–28 weeks if first one normal.
Counselling points		• Women with GDM have an increased risk of developing T2DM later in life. Therefore, dietary changes should be encouraged to continue, and annual monitoring with HbA1c.

TABLE 11.14

Pre-Existing Diabetes (T1DM and T2DM)

Antenatal	Extra tests	• Test fasting, 1 hour post meal and bedtime blood glucose levels daily (although continuous glucose monitoring is preferable) • Target levels; fasting <5.3, 1 hour post meal <7.8, 2-hour post meal <6.4 • T1DM should keep blood glucose level >4 • Test for ketonaemia if hyperglycaemic/unwell • Retinal assessment at booking and 28/40 (plus at 16– 20/40 if they have diabetic retinopathy) • Renal assessment at booking if not done in last three months. Refer if creatinine >120, urinary albumin:creatinine ratio (uACR) >30. Thromboprophylaxis if ACR >220 (nephrotic range). • Joint diabetic clinic 1–2 weekly
	Extra scans	• Serial USS 28–40/40
	Delivery	• If uncomplicated – plan delivery 37–38+6. • Consider <37/40 if metabolic/maternal/fetal complications. • Diabetic retinopathy is a contraindication to vaginal birth.
Intrapartum	Increased risk/prophylaxis for increased risk	• If requiring antenatal steroids – risk of hyperglycaemia – admit for BM monitoring and give additional insulin/ sliding scale depending on BMs. • Monitor BMs hourly during labour, target range 4–7 mmol/L. • Consider sliding scale from onset of labour in T1DM.
	Monitoring in labour	cEFM
Postnatal		• Reduce insulin to pre-pregnancy dose (unless diabetes had been poorly controlled prior). • Risk of hypoglycaemia if breastfeeding. • Metformin and insulin safe whilst breastfeeding, other oral blood-glucose lowering therapy is not. • Baby will need blood glucose monitoring for at least 24 hours post birth. • Encourage woman to feed baby within 30 minutes, and then 2–3 hourly.
Counselling points		• Importance of pre-pregnancy counselling in future pregnancies to ensure optimisation prior to conception

TABLE 11.15

Large for Gestational Age (LGA)

Antenatal	Extra tests	• GTT if not previously performed • Serial fundal height measurements following diagnosis of LGA to ensure normal trajectory being followed.
	Extra scans	• LGA diagnosed if EFW >90th centile on customised growth chart.
	Delivery	• Options; expectant management, IOL, elective LSCS • IOL reduces risk of shoulder dystocia from 20:1000 to 7:1000 but increases risk of 3rd/4th degree tears from 6:1000 to 29:1000. No difference in perinatal death, brachial plexus injury or need for emergency LSCS. • Recommend elective LSCS if EFW ≥5kg.
Intrapartum	Increased risk/prophylaxis for increased risk	Risk of shoulder dystocia: • CLC if EFW >97th centile on USS • Otherwise, can choose setting, including water birth (but explain to woman that she may be asked to get out if there are concerns). • Senior review if delay in first stage, prior to commencing oxytocin • Early recourse to LSCS if no descent of presenting part. • Instrumental delivery should be performed in theatre.
	Monitoring in labour	• Intermittent auscultation (IA) if no other risk factors present.
Postnatal		• Risk PPH – recommend active management of 3rd stage.
Future pregnancies		• If shoulder dystocia occurs, risk of shoulder dystocia in future pregnancy is increased. If brachial plexus injury occurs, elective LSCS is recommended in future pregnancies.
Counselling points		• Ultrasound scans have a 10% margin of error (therefore significantly more in an LGA baby) and a sensitivity of 50%–60% for macrosomia. • Half of cases of shoulder dystocia occur in babies <4 kg. • Brachial plexus injury following shoulder dystocia is rare.

TABLE 11.16

Small for Gestational Age (SGA)

Antenatal	Extra tests	• If severe SGA at anomaly scan, refer for detailed anatomical scan and UAD by fetal med. • If severe SGA <23/40 or anomalies detected, offer karyotyping. • Screen for CMV and toxoplasmosis in severe SGA. • Test for syphilis and malaria in high-risk populations. • Encourage smoking cessation if relevant.
	Extra scans	• Abdominal circumference (AC) or EFW <10th centile is diagnostic of SGA. • <3rd centile is severe SGA (plotted on a customised growth chart). • 2-weekly serial USS for EFW and UAD following diagnosis of SGA (if UAD is normal). • More frequent Doppler surveillance if severe SGA.
	Delivery	• Timing depending on Doppler indices. (Refer to algorithm in RCOG 2023, Greentop guideline 31.) • Can offer IOL if normal UAD/raised PI but EDF present (but increased rate of LSCS). • If absent or reversed end diastolic volume (AREDV), for LSCS.
Intrapartum	Increased risk/prophylaxis for increased risk	• Risk of prematurity if early delivery (more likely in an SGA fetus) • Offer antenatal corticosteroids if delivery planned <36/40 • MgSO$_4$ if in established labour <34/40 or having planned preterm birth <34/40
	Monitoring in labour	• cEFM from onset of contractions. (Women should be advised to attend early in labour to allow commencement of cEFM.)
Postnatal		• Nothing specific to SGA baby.
Future pregnancies		• Previous SGA is a major risk factor for SGA in next pregnancy (2x increased risk). • Serial USS for EFW and UAD from 26–28/40. • Start aspirin 150mg ON from 12/40.
Counselling points		

TABLE 11.17

In Vitro Fertilization (IVF) Pregnancy

Antenatal	Extra tests	• Overall, IVF pregnancy should be managed as per a spontaneous pregnancy, but with an awareness of the small increased risks. • A thorough risk assessment is imperative, as many women undergoing ART have additional risk factors that will necessitate increased monitoring. • ART alone is **not** an indication for GTT, aspirin or low-molecular-weight heparin (LMWH) in the absence of other risk factors. • For combined screening, use age of egg donor if donor eggs have been used in IVF.
	Extra scans	• Serial USS only if other risk factors present. (Women may request for reassurance.) • If low-lying placenta at anomaly scan, TV USS with colour Doppler to exclude vasa praevia.
	Delivery	• Consider IOL at term (increased risk of SB). • Increased likelihood of maternal choice elective LSCS.
Intrapartum	Increased risk/prophylaxis for increased risk	• No increased intrapartum risks specifically related to IVF. • Awareness that maternal anxiety likely to be high and so sufficient support should be provided in labour.
	Monitoring in labour	• Based on risk assessment. • Some women will request cEFM for peace of mind; others will request as little intervention as possible.
Postnatal		• Inform women of chance of spontaneous conception even following IVF pregnancy.
Future pregnancies		• Nil specific following IVF pregnancy.
Counselling points		• IVF pregnancies carry a **small** increased risk of perinatal mortality, preterm birth, low birth weight, NICU admission, placenta praevia, GDM, and PET. • Some evidence of increased risk of fetal structural abnormalities.

TABLE 11.18

Previous Intra-Uterine Death

Antenatal	Extra tests	• **Pre-conception** – offer general advice such as smoking cessation, healthy diet, weight loss (if BMI >25), psychological support. (Discuss potential benefit of delaying conception until severe psychological issues resolved.) • **Next pregnancy** – clear documentation of history in notes to be read thoroughly by anyone seeing patient. • CLC, GTT
	Extra scans	• Serial USS if previous SGA (although woman may request serial USS for reassurance).
	Delivery	• Previous unexplained intrauterine fetal demise (IUFD) is indication for consultant-led delivery. • If previous IUFD due to known nonrecurrent cause, individualise assessment re place of birth. • Individualised discussion re scheduled birth after discussion with consultant.
Intrapartum	Increased risk/prophylaxis for increased risk	• Increased risk of intrapartum stillbirth following previous unexplained IUFD. • Other risks depend on factors in current pregnancy – manage accordingly.
	Monitoring in labour	• cEFM most common practice (if previous IUFD due to known non-recurrent cause, and no additional risk factors this pregnancy, can have IA if this is the preference of the woman).
Postnatal		• Bonding may be adversely affected. • High risk of PND – partner and support network should be aware of signs.
Future pregnancies		• As above – be mindful that irrespective of a subsequent delivery of a healthy baby, all future pregnancies/ deliveries following an IUD are likely to be a source of distress. As such, remain vigilant for difficulties with bonding or signs of post-natal depression (PND).
Counselling points		• Women who stop smoking have equivalent stillbirth rates to women who have never smoked. • No evidence that routine IOL following previous IUFD improves outcomes for baby but increases rate of operative delivery. (However, this may be outweighed by psychological benefit to the woman, so individualised discussion is always warranted.)

TABLE 11.19

Vaginal Birth after Caesarean (VBAC)

Antenatal	Extra tests	• Full history detailing previous C/S and identify any risk factors which would be a contraindication to VBAC this time (classical incision, short inter– pregnancy interval). • Discussion and completion of VBAC decision making tools which are often available in local guidelines.
	Extra scans	• If anterior low-lying placenta, consider MRI to rule out invasive placenta.
	Delivery	• Aim for spontaneous labour; consider stretch and sweep from 38 weeks to increase chance of spontaneous labour. • Senior review if IOL indicated (increased risk of scar dehiscence/LSCS) – mechanical methods carry lower risk.

Intrapartum	Increased risk/prophylaxis for increased risk	• Risk of scar dehiscence/rupture (0.2%–0.5% risk)
		  • CLC delivery with resources for emergency LSCS if concerns.
		  • IV access, FBC and valid G+S.
		  • Beware of sudden increase in analgesia requirements, especially if pain persisting between contractions and/or over scar.
		  • Minimum 4-hourly vaginal examination – slowing of progress or loss of station of presenting part.
		  • Observe for abnormal vaginal bleeding.
		  • Observe for haematuria.

	Monitoring in labour	• cEFM from onset of contractions.
Postnatal		• Nil specific for VBAC.
Future pregnancies		• Following successful VBAC, chance of successful vaginal delivery in future pregnancies rises to 85%–90%. • Will still require individualised discussion regarding MOD next pregnancy.
Counselling points		• See example of VBAC decision-making tool for main counselling points.

TABLE 11.20

Preterm Prelabour Rupture of Membranes (PPROM)

Antenatal	Extra tests	• Speculum to confirm PPROM (+ test of vaginal fluid if no obvious liquor seen). • Blood test for inflammatory markers. • CTG for fetal well-being. • Admit for monitoring for 24–48 h. Can then be monitored as outpatient if no signs of infection or labour. Follow-up as per individual unit protocol (usually 1–2x per week). • Inform neonatal team if delivery anticipated.
	Extra scans	• May be required to monitor fetal growth if early PPROM.
	Delivery	• Conservative Mx until 37/40, and then offer IOL. • Consider earlier delivery if signs of chorioamnionitis. • GBS carriers – commence antibiotics at onset of labour. Consider IOL from 34/40.
Intrapartum	Increased risk/prophylaxis for increased risk	• Risk of infection – commence erythromycin 250 mg four times a day (QDS) for 10/7 (or until established labour). • Temperature monitoring QDS (by woman if O/P). • Antenatal corticosteroids depending on gestation. • $MgSO_4$ if in established labour or having planned preterm birth <34/40. • Do not give tocolysis to women with PPROM.
	Monitoring in labour	• cEFM advised. Fetal tachycardia may indicate infection – low threshold to deliver.
Postnatal		• If raised inflammatory markers, monitor until stable/improving prior to discharge. • Consider continuing abx based on clinical picture and blood results. • Neonatal review of baby.
Future pregnancies		• Under care of obstetrician with interest in preterm birth. • 8x risk recurrence PPROM next pregnancy.
Counselling points		• Median duration of pregnancy after PPROM is seven days and shortens as gestation advances. • Clinical signs of infection to observe for – lower abdominal pain, abnormal PV discharge, fever, malaise, reduced fetal movements [RFMs]).

TABLE 11.21

Preterm Labour and Threatened Preterm Labour (PTL/TPTL)

Antenatal	Extra tests	• Speculum examination (+/– digital VE if unable to visualise cervix with a speculum).
		• USS for cervical length if >30/40
		  • CL >15mm – reassure unlikely PTL
		  • CL <15mm – diagnose PTL
		• Alternative test such as fetal fibronectin if USS not available

	Extra scans	• Cervical length scan • Scan for EFW
	Delivery	• Consider augmentation if PPROM with signs of infection • Consider LSCS if breech
Intrapartum	Increased risk/prophylaxis for increased risk	• Risks of prematurity. Consider rescue cerclage if dilated cervix and exposed, unruptured membranes 16–28/40 (not if contracting). • Nifedipine tocolysis can be used 24–34/40 to facilitate intra-uterine transfer and/or administration of steroids (avoid tocolysis if PPROM or signs of bleeding). • Antenatal corticosteroids should be considered and discussed 24–34/40. • $MgSO_4$ for fetal neuroprotection <34/40. • Offer intrapartum antibiotics from diagnosis of labour until birth of baby.
	Monitoring in labour	• cEFM advised in most cases (unless PTL at pre-viable gestation). • Care with using FSE <34/40. • IA can be considered if no other risk factors – no evidence that it alters outcome.
Postnatal		• Neonatal input for baby • Emotional support for parents
Future pregnancies		• Referral to preterm birth clinic. • Patients with previous PTB <34/40 should be offered vaginal progesterone and should receive 2– weekly cervical length USS from 16– 24/40 (if <25mm then offer either vaginal progesterone or prophylactic cervical cerclage).
Counselling points		• Emergency cerclage aims to delay birth, increase likelihood of baby surviving and reduce senior neonatal morbidity.

TABLE 11.22

Minor Antepartum Haemorrhage (APH)

Antenatal	Extra tests	• Full examination and observations • Speculum examination (caution if known low-lying placenta) • Bloods – FBC, G+S, Kleihauer (if Rh–ve) • Anti-D if Rh–ve (in recurrent APH, at least 6-weekly doses should be given). • cCTG • Admit any woman with ongoing bleeding/CTG concerns.
	Extra scans	• USS for placental localisation if no recent scan • Serial USS for fetal growth following recurrent minor APH (unless proven from ectropion/lower genital tract).
	Delivery	• Consider IOL at term following recurrent APH in pregnancy.

Intrapartum	Increased risk/prophylaxis for increased risk	• Risk of preterm birth and associated risks prematurity
		  • Consider MgSO$_4$ if delivery expected <34/40
		  • Consider steroids if delivery expected 24– 34+6/40
		• Risk massive APH
		  • Ensure valid G+S, and XM blood available

	Monitoring in labour	• cEFM in most cases (except after one minor APH with no subsequent fetal concerns).
Postnatal		• Increased risk of PPH – active 3rd stage advised (Syntometrine if no contraindications). • Consider thromboprophylaxis (haemorrhage and blood transfusion are risk factors for venous thromboembolism [VTE]). • Neonatal involvement if bleeding ongoing in labour.
Future pregnancies		
Counselling points		• First trimester bleeding slightly increases risk of abruption in later pregnancy (from 1%–1.4%). • Modify known risk factors – smoking, cocaine and amphetamine use. • Consider possibility of domestic violence as cause for APH.

TABLE 11.23

Major Antepartum Haemorrhage (APH)

Antenatal	Extra tests	• Stabilise woman if maternal compromise – involve anaesthetist. • Full examination and observations. • Speculum examination (caution if known low-lying placenta) • Bloods – FBC, G+S, Kleihauer (if Rh−ve), plus coagulation, U+Es, LFTs and XM 4 units. • cCTG • Activate major haemorrhage protocol if appropriate.
	Extra scans	• Bedside USS to confirm placental location if planning LSCS. • If bleeding resolves/not for immediate delivery, then perform USS for fetal well-being.
	Delivery	• Urgent LSCS if maternal/fetal compromise, following stabilisation (consider GA to aid maternal resuscitation and expedite delivery). • If IUFD is diagnosed and woman is stable, vaginal birth is recommended.

Intrapartum	Increased risk/prophylaxis for increased risk	• Risk of preterm birth and associated risks prematurity
		  • Consider $MgSO_4$ if delivery expected <34/40
		  • Consider steroids if delivery expected 24–34+6/40
		• Risk massive APH
		  • Ensure valid G+S, and XM blood available
		  • Major haemorrhage protocol
		  • High likelihood of needing blood transfusion
		• Risk disseminated intravascular (DIC) in massive ongoing bleeding
		  • Monitor platelets and ensure adequate clotting factors being replaced.
		  • Involve haematologist.
		  • Up to 4 units FFP and 10 units cryoprecipitate can be given in relentless bleeding whilst awaiting results of clotting studies.

	Monitoring in labour	• cEFM
Postnatal		• Increased risk of PPH – active 3rd stage advised (Syntometrine if no contraindications). • Consider thromboprophylaxis (haemorrhage and blood transfusion are risk factors for VTE). • Neonatal involvement – prematurity, hyperbilirubinaemia, low birth weight all risks. • Thorough debriefing of patient, partners and staff.
Future pregnancies		• If APH due to placental abruption, risk of recurrence in future pregnancies (4.4% if one previous abruption, up to 25% if two previous abruptions).

TABLE 11.24

Post-Dates Pregnancy (>41/40)

Antenatal	Extra tests	• Discuss options of expectant management versus LSCS. • For expectant management, offer additional fetal monitoring (twice-weekly CTG and USS for liquor volume [LV]). Advise woman that this monitoring only gives a snapshot of baby's well-being, and adverse events such as stillbirth cannot be reliably predicted or prevented even with monitoring.
	Extra scans	• USS at 40/40 if required serial USS throughout pregnancy • Twice-weekly USS for LV.
	IOL	• Immediate IOL should be offered if the woman changes her mind at any point.
Intrapartum	Increased risk/prophylaxis for increased risk	• Increased risk SB/neonatal death beyond 42/40 – for cEFM in labour.
	Monitoring in labour	• cEFM advised
Postnatal		• Nil specific for post-dates, but awareness of potential co-existing factors such as large baby, long labour, which may predispose to PPH.
Future pregnancies		• Nil relevant for future pregnancies.
Counselling points		• Risks associated with pregnancy beyond 41/40; increased chance LSCS, increased chance NICU admission for baby, increased risk of SB and neonatal death. These risks are further increased in women who are black or from other ethnic minorities, or from more deprived areas.

Note: NICE (2021) advises IOL for uncomplicated pregnancies between 41 and 42/40. This table covers management of women who decline IOL.

TABLE 11.25

Polyhydramnios

Antenatal	Extra tests		• GTT, TORCH screen. • Check maternal blood group and consider Kleihauer if Rh–ve and suspicion of FMH/fetal anaemia. • Drug history – lithium can lead to fetal diabetes insipidus (and increased fetal urine output). • CTG if concerns with RFMs. • Consider admission if severe polyhydramnios and high presenting part/non-cephalic presentation. • Refer to fetal medicine if suspected fetal anomaly, SGA, severe polyhydramnios.
	Extra scans		• Polyhydramnios defined when DVP ≥8 cm on USS (moderate if 12–15 cm, severe if ≥16 cm • Repeat USS after two weeks to monitor liquor volume • Detailed fetal USS to rule out any organ anomalies or tumours (more likely with severe polyhydramnios)
	Delivery		• IOL at 39–40/40 if DVP > 12cm
Intrapartum	Increased risk/prophylaxis for increased risk		• Risk cord prolapse if high presenting part – for controlled ARM during IOL. • Risk placental abruption if rapid uterine decompression – controlled ARM
	Monitoring in labour		• cEFM advised due to risk of cord prolapse
Postnatal			• Risk PPH – advise active management of third stage. • Inform neonatal team of delivery – need to consider passing NG tube after birth.
Future pregnancies			• Risk of recurrence only if underlying cause of polyhydramnios found
Counselling points			• Advise TCI ASAP if SROM due to risk cord prolapse. • Polyhydramnios carries increased risk of PPROM, PTB, cord prolapse, NICU admission, PPH and need for LSCS.

TABLE 11.26

Oligohydramnios

Antenatal	Extra tests		• History +/– speculum examination to rule out ruptured membranes • BP to rule out PET as a cause. • Medication review (ACE inhibitors [ACEi] and non-steroidal anti-inflammatory drugs [NSAIDs] can be cause). • Consider karyotyping (likely fetal medicine decision), particularly if early unexplained oligohydramnios.
	Extra scans		• USS demonstrating DVP ≤2 cm is diagnostic of oligohydramnios (or AFI <5th centile for gestational age). • USS for EFW as often associated with SGA (add UAD if EFW <10th centile) • Fetal anomaly scan if not already done (to r/o fetal renal pathology). • Repeat EFW/LV/UAD every two weeks if stable.
	Delivery		• Consider IOL 37–38 weeks • Senior review if associated SGA/ intrauterine growth restriction (IUGR) as earlier delivery may be indicated. • Consider LSCS if anhydramnios
Intrapartum	Increased risk/prophylaxis for increased risk		• Risk umbilical cord compression and meconium aspiration during labour – for cEFM. • Anhydramnios – risk of fetal deformation due to compression effects – for referral to fetal medicine specialist.
	Monitoring in labour		• cEFM advised
Postnatal			• Neonatal involvement, especially if associated IUGR
Future pregnancies			• May be risk of recurrence depending on underlying cause • For unexplained oligohydramnios, no evidence of recurrence in future pregnancies
Counselling points			• Dx of oligohydramnios in second trimester more likely to be associated with fetal or maternal anomalies; diagnosis in third trimester more likely to be unexplained origin.

TABLE 11.27

Low-Lying Placenta and Placenta Praevia

Antenatal	Extra tests	• Regular G+S to ensure valid result always available in case of haemorrhage. • Regular FBC and prompt management of anaemia • If asymptomatic, counsel re risk of PTB and haemorrhage, ensure they have a way to attend hospital immediately if needed. • Admit any woman with bleeding
	Extra scans	• Usually identified at anomaly scan – placenta praevia if covering internal os, low-lying placenta if <20mm from internal os. • Follow-up USS at 32/40 (TVUS improves accuracy of placental localisation) • If persistent at 32/40, USS again at 36/40 (90% will have resolved by term). • Cervical length scanning can be considered – CL <25 mm is risk for major obstetric haemorrhage (MOH) during LSCS.
	Delivery	• 34–36+6 if bleeding in pregnancy or other risk factors for PTB • 36–37/40 if uncomplicated • LSCS for all women with known placenta praevia or low-lying placenta

Intrapartum	Increased risk/prophylaxis for increased risk	• Risk PTB (spontaneous and iatrogenic)
		  • Consider steroids <35+6/50.
		  • $MgSO_4$ <34/40.
		  • Tocolysis can be considered to aid administration of the above.
		• Risk of massive haemorrhage
		  • Discuss risk blood transfusion and hysterectomy (include on consent form).
		  • Cell salvage should be used and a rapid infuser available.
		  • Use USS to confirm placental location and avoid incising through placenta wherever possible.
		  • Vertical incision if baby in transverse lie, particularly <28/40 (to avoid placenta).
		  • If placenta is incised, immediate cord clamping is indicated.
		  • Early recourse to intrauterine tamponade/surgical haemostatic techniques/interventional radiology (IR).
		  • Early recourse to hysterectomy if medical/surgical techniques are ineffective.

Postnatal		• Risk of PPH • Thromboprophylaxis once bleeding has settled.
Future pregnancies		• Risk of placenta praevia increased in future pregnancies, particularly following repeated LSCS (10:1000 with one previous LSCS, 28:1000 with 3+ previous LSCS). • Increased risk if subsequent pregnancy <1 year following LSCS.
Counselling points		• Risk factors for LLP/placenta praevia; previous LSCS (risk increases with higher number of previous LSCS), ART, maternal smoking.

TABLE 11.28

Placenta Accreta Spectrum (PAS)

Antenatal	Extra tests	• If PAS diagnosed, care should be in specialist centre, including delivery. • A contingency plan for emergency delivery should be in place.
	Extra scans	• Women with previous LSCS and anterior low-lying placenta, or placenta praevia are at high risk – refer for USS by a specialist in diagnosing invasive placentas. • MRI not needed as routine but can complement USS by assessing depth/lateral extension of invasion.
	Delivery	• LSCS at 35–36+6/40 if otherwise uncomplicated • Individualised discussion if other risk factors for PTB present

Intrapartum	Increased risk/prophylaxis for increased risk	• Risk massive haemorrhage
		  • Cell salvage, availability of blood products, medical/surgical/IR intervention
		• High risk of hysterectomy.
		  • Caesarean hysterectomy with placenta left *in situ* is preferable to attempting to separate placenta from uterine wall (apart from some specific circumstances and by expert teams).
		  • Expectant management can be considered in some circumstances whereby the placenta is left *in situ*.
		• Risk lower urinary tract damage.
		• A consent form specific to LSCS for PAS should cover the above risks.

Postnatal		• Risk PPH • Thromboprophylaxis (massive haemorrhage and blood transfusion are risk factors) • Regular follow-up via USS (and access to emergency care) if placenta has been left *in situ*. • Postnatal debriefing is essential.
Future pregnancies		• If uterus is preserved, careful counselling regarding increased risk in future pregnancies and future C/S.
Counselling points		• Major risk factors are hx of placenta accreta, previous LSCS (increasing risk with increasing no. of previous LSCS) and repeated endometrial curettage. • In women with placenta praevia and previous LSCS, risk of PAS is; 3%, 11%, 40%, 61% and 67% for one, two, three, four and five previous LSCS, respectively.

TABLE 11.29

Vasa Praevia

Antenatal	Extra tests	• Antenatal diagnosis improves fetal survival from 40% to over 95%. • Painless vaginal bleeding following SROM/ARM should alert to possibility of vasa praevia, and immediate delivery should be facilitated. • Individualise discussion regarding hospitalisation from 32/40.
	Extra scans	• Diagnosed using a combination of TA and TV colour Doppler imaging USS (although routine screening for vasa praevia currently not indicated). • Confirm persistence of vasa praevia by USS in the third trimester.
	Delivery	• El LSCS at 34–36 weeks in asymptomatic women
Intrapartum	Increased risk/prophylaxis for increased risk	• With ruptured vasa praevia, blood being lost is fetal blood, and so a relatively small amount of blood can quickly result in complete fetal exsanguination. • Risk of iatrogenic prematurity: • Steroids if planned delivery <36/40 • $MgSO_4$ if planned delivery <34/40
Postnatal		• Paediatric involvement imperative. • Send placenta for histology if vasa praevia diagnosed when stillbirth or acute fetal compromise has occurred.
Future pregnancies		• No evidence of increased risk in future pregnancies.
Counselling points		• When deciding whether prophylactic hospital admission from 32/40 is appropriate, factors to consider include multiple pregnancy, antenatal bleeding and risk factors for preterm labour.

Bibliography

Alfirevic Z et al. Continuous cardiotocography (CTG) as a form of electronic fetal monitoring (EFM) for fetal assessment during labour. Cochrane Database Syst Rev. 2017;2(2):CD006066.

Cluett ER et al. Immersion in water during labour and birth. Cochrane Database Syst Rev. 2018;5(5):CD000111.

Dominguez-Bello MG et al. Delivery mode shapes the acquisition and structure of the initial microbiota across multiple body habitats in newborns. Proc Natl Acad Sci USA. 2010;107(26):11971–5.

Johanson RB, Menon BK. Vacuum extraction versus forceps for assisted vaginal delivery. Cochrane Database Syst Rev. 2000;2(2):CD000224.

Khalife N et al. Prenatal glucocorticoid treatment and later mental health in children and adolescents. PLoS One. 2013;8(11):e81394.

National Institute for Health and Care Excellence. Intrapartum care [Internet]. [London]. NICE; 2008 (Clinical guideline [NG235]).

National Institute for Health and Care Excellence. Hypertension in pregnancy [Internet]. [London]. NICE; 2010 (Clinical guideline [CG107]).

National Institute for Health and Care Excellence. Intrapartum care [Internet]. [London]. NICE; 2014 (Clinical guideline [NG235]).

National Institute for Health and Care Excellence. Preterm labour and birth [Internet]. [London]. NICE; 2015 (Clinical guideline [NG25]).

National Institute for Health and Care Excellence. Intrapartum care for women with existing medical conditions or obstetric complications and their babies [Internet]. [London]. NICE; 2019 (Clinical guideline [NG121]).

National Institute for Health and Care Excellence. Caesarean birth [Internet]. [London]. NICE; 2021a (Clinical guideline [NG192]).

National Institute for Health and Care Excellence. Inducing labour [Internet]. [London]. NICE; 2021b (Clinical guideline [NG207]).

National Institute for Health and Care Excellence. Intrapartum care [Internet]. [London]. NICE; 2023 (Clinical guideline [NG235]).

PROMPT Maternity Foundation. PROMPT Course Manual. Cambridge University Press; 2012.

Royal College of Obstetricians and Gynaecologists. Antepartum haemorrhage [Internet]. [London]. RCOG; 2011a (Green-top guideline no. 63).

Royal College of Obstetricians and Gynaecologists. Care of women with obesity in pregnancy [Internet]. [London]. RCOG; 2011b (Green-top guideline no. 72).

Royal College of Obstetricians and Gynaecologists. Chicken pox in pregnancy [Internet]. [London]. RCOG; 2011c (Green-top guideline no. 13).

Royal College of Obstetricians and Gynaecologists. Bacterial sepsis following pregnancy [Internet]. [London]. RCOG; 2012a (Green-top guideline no. 64b).

Royal College of Obstetricians and Gynaecologists. Sepsis in pregnancy [Internet]. [London]. RCOG; 2012b (Green-top guideline no. 64a).

Royal College of Obstetricians and Gynaecologists. Umbilical cord prolapse [Internet]. [London]. RCOG; 2014a (Green-top guideline no. 50).

Royal College of Obstetricians and Gynaecologists. Perinatal management of pregnant women at the threshold of infant. Viability (The Obstetric Perspective) [Internet]. [London]. RCOG; 2014b (RCOG Scientific Impact Paper no. 41).

Royal College of Obstetricians and Gynaecologists. Birth after previous caesarean section [Internet]. [London]. RCOG; 2015a (Green-top guideline no. 45).

Royal College of Obstetricians and Gynaecologists. Antepartum haemorrhage [Internet]. [London]. RCOG; 2015b (Green-top guideline no. 47).

Royal College of Obstetricians and Gynaecologists. Reducing the risk of thrombosis and embolism during pregnancy and the puerperium [Internet]. [London]. RCOG; 2015c (Green-top guideline no. 37a).

Royal College of Obstetricians and Gynaecologists. Third- and fourth- degree perineal tears, management [Internet]. [London]. RCOG; 2015d (Green-top guideline no. 29).

Royal College of Obstetricians and Gynaecologists. Prevention and management of post-partum haemorrhage [Internet]. [London]. RCOG; 2016 (Green-top guideline no. 52).

Royal College of Obstetricians and Gynaecologists. External cephalic version and reducing the incidence of term breech presentation [Internet]. [London]. RCOG; 2017a (Green-top guideline no. 20a).

Royal College of Obstetricians and Gynaecologists. Management of breech presentation [Internet]. [London]. RCOG; 2017b (Green-top guideline no. 20b).

Royal College of Obstetricians and Gynaecologists. Prevention of early-onset group B streptococcal disease [Internet]. [London]. RCOG; 2017c (Green-top guideline no. 36).

Royal College of Obstetricians and Gynaecologists. Placenta praevia and placenta praevia accreta: Diagnosis and management [Internet]. [London]. RCOG; 2018a (Green-top guideline no. 27a).

Royal College of Obstetricians and Gynaecologists. Vasa praevia: Diagnosis and management [Internet]. [London]. RCOG; 2018b (Green-top guideline no. 27b).

Royal College of Obstetricians and Gynaecologists. Care of women presenting with suspected preterm prelabour rupture of membranes from 24+0 weeks of gestation [Internet]. [London]. RCOG; 2019a (Green-top guideline no. 73).

Royal College of Obstetricians and Gynaecologists. Maternal collapse in pregnancy and the puerperium [Internet]. [London]. RCOG; 2019b (Green-top guideline no. 56).

Royal College of Obstetricians and Gynaecologists. Assisted vaginal birth [Internet]. [London]. RCOG; 2020 (Green-top guideline no. 26).

Royal College of Obstetricians and Gynaecologists. Antenatal corticosteroids to reduce neonatal morbidity and mortality [Internet]. [London]. RCOG; 2022a (Green-top guideline no. 74).

Royal College of Obstetricians and Gynaecologists. Cervical cerclage [Internet]. [London]. RCOG; 2022b (Green-top guideline no. 75).

Royal College of Obstetricians and Gynaecologists. Intrahepatic cholestasis of pregnancy [Internet]. [London]. RCOG; 2022c (Green-top guideline no. 43).

Royal College of Obstetricians and Gynaecologists. Planned caesarean birth [Internet]. [London]. RCOG; 2022d (RCOG consent advice no. 14).

Royal College of Obstetricians and Gynaecologists. Investigation and care of a small-for gestational-age fetus and growth restricted fetus. [Internet]. [London]. RVOG; 2023 (Green-top guideline no. 31)

Royal College of Obstetricians and Gynaecologists. Care of late intrauterine fetal death and stillbirth [Internet]. [London]. RCOG; 2024a (Green-top guideline no. 55).

Royal College of Obstetricians and Gynaecologists. Small-for-gestational age fetus and growth restricted fetus investigation and care [Internet]. [London]. RCOG; 2024b (Green-top guideline no. 31).

Royal College of Obstetricians and Gynaecologists and British Association of Sexual Health and HIV Joint Guideline. Genital herpes in pregnancy, management [Internet]. [London]: BASSH; 2024.

Royal College of Obstetricians and Gynaecologists and British HIV Society. HIV in pregnancy, management [Internet]. [London]: BHIVA; 2018 (Green-top guideline no. 39).

Royal College of Obstetricians and Gynaecologists and UK Haemophilia Centre Doctor's Organisation Joint Guidelines. Management of inherited bleeding disorders in pregnancy [Internet]. [London]. RCOG/UKHCDO; 2017 (Green-top guideline no. 71).

Thomas J et al. The national sentinel caesarean section audit. BJOG. 2000;107(5):579–80.

Index

Note: Locators in *italics* represent figures and **bold** indicate tables in the text.